MW01679294

IN THE JUNGLE OF MEDICINE:
Journeys Through Caribbean Medical School

Dr. Tiffany Bursey
Dr. Vanessa Doyle
Dr. Hedieh Ghanbari
Dr. Raheleh Sarbaziha

IN THE JUNGLE OF MEDICINE: Journeys through Caribbean Medical School

ISBN 978-1-63263-121-3

Published by BookLocker.com, Inc., Bradenton, Florida.

Printed in the United States of America.

BookLocker.com, Inc.
2014

First Edition

Dr. Tiffany Bursey
Dr. Vanessa Doyle
Dr. Hedieh Ghanbari
Dr. Raheleh Sarbaziha

DEDICATION

We wish to offer a special thank you to our parents, spouses, partners, and all those people who believed in us as we journeyed through the jungle of medicine. Your love and support shall never be forgotten. Never!

And to our children and future children who will come to know their moms as trailblazers who defied the odds. May you light the future trail even brighter!

A special thank you to our incredible editors: Chuck & Carley. Your dedication to making this book a reality can never be repaid. Thank you, thank you and thank you again!

And to those who are coming behind us: the dream is possible if the will is there.

Finally we dedicate this book to the people of Dominica who allowed us to share their beautiful country for one brief shining moment in our medical journeys.

A percentage of the commissions from all sales of this book will be donated to Princess Margaret Hospital in Roseau Dominica.

T V H & R

DISCLAIMER

This book details the author's personal experiences with and opinions about Caribbean medical school..

The author and publisher are providing this book and its contents on an "as is" basis and make no representations or warranties of any kind with respect to this book or its contents. The author and publisher disclaim all such representations and warranties, including for example warranties of merchantability and any advice for a particular purpose. In addition, the author and publisher do not represent or warrant that the information accessible via this book is accurate, complete or current.

The statements made about products and services the U.S. government has not evaluated. Please consult with your own legal or accounting professional regarding the suggestions and recommendations made in this book.

Except as specifically stated in this book, neither the author or publisher, nor any authors, contributors, or other representatives will be liable for damages arising out of or in connection with the use of this book. This is a comprehensive limitation of liability that applies to all damages of any kind, including (without limitation) compensatory; direct, indirect or consequential damages; loss of data, income or profit; loss of or damage to property and claims of third parties.

You understand that this book is not intended as a substitute for consultation with a licensed medical, legal or accounting professional. Before you begin any change your lifestyle in any way, you will consult a licensed professional to ensure that you are doing what's best for your situation.

This book provides content related to the study of medicine in the Caribbean and other topics. As such, use of this book implies your acceptance of this disclaimer.

TABLE OF CONTENTS

What people are saying about IN THE JUNGLE OF MEDICINE

Having taught medicine in Canada (McMaster) and in the Caribbean (Ross) I can personally attest to the great differences between the academic and philosophical approach to learning medicine in Canada and at a US Caribbean medical school. Living abroad can be extremely stressful and when you add this to the normal stressors of medical school one can understand how motivated one has to be to become a physician if one chooses the Caribbean route. You are forever an IMG (International Medical Graduate) and the extra maze of paperwork that has to be done is daunting. While not exactly a vade mecum, I think the experiences of these four Canadians who studied medicine abroad will help inform any Canadian who is contemplating studying in the Caribbean or is even already there and wondering whether they are unique in their frustrations and difficulties about what it is really like. Being well informed before one takes the huge step may decrease the shock on arrival. The comfort of knowing that despite the difficulties one can get through and out the other side is priceless. The practical information appended about examinations, getting a residency will save you a great deal of time and may well help you get back home to practice, like these four fantastic doctors who show what can be done if you persist and believe; which is what it's all about.

Anne White MD FRCPC
(Retired Professor of Medicine)

It's nice to have somebody finally put some real and personal perspective on "off shore" medical schools especially Ross University School of Medicine. People need to understand the journey these people go through is very tough and the notion of medical school under the sun is far from the truth. These successful doctors are determined and had a dream to fulfill and achieved their goals. Where there is a will there is a way!!

Ali Novin MD
PGY - 4 University of Toronto

For anyone who has ever considered studying medicine in the Caribbean or has wondered what life is like for a Caribbean med student...this is a must read. Anyone who would leave the country they love, without the guarantee of returning, is fully committed to the study and practice of medicine. Catch a glimpse into the "med school boot camp" that is the island, and see what challenges and triumphs shape some of the worlds' most globally minded, socially aware and highly effective doctors in our society today.

Rachelle Krause
Hons BSc (UOIT), MS4 (RUSM)

This book is the perfect roadmap for students thinking of attending a Caribbean medical school. There was no such map when I attended medical school in the Caribbean and it can be a lonely journey with no direction. The authors are to be commended for telling their stories in such a moving and honest way. Studying in a Caribbean medical school is no cakewalk. I know, I did it. Read the book for pleasure and for a deeper understanding of what motivates a person to go to the tropics, study medicine and come home having truly earned the right to be called Doctor!

Dr. Michael Van Vliet (B.PE, B.Ed, MD, CCFP, EM Fellowship)
Emergency Room Physician
UBC Clinical Professor

It's a scary prospect leaving your home country to study medicine in a foreign land. You learn a lot about yourself, your limitations, and your priorities. These four incredible doctors are opening a huge window into this frightening and exhilarating adventure that could lie ahead. This book is both a guidepost for future students and a treasure of memories for those of us who have shared in this amazing journey.

Ida Cavaliere, MD
(PGY 1 University of Toronto)

Navigating the perils of medical school in a foreign land is an intimidating endeavor. Moreover, moving forward in your career as an IMG presents many collective and unique personal challenges. Only those who go through the process can truly understand this. The strength of this book lies in the fact that these are former students who actually went through this arduous process. This book courageously outlines the journey through personal experience and anecdotal storytelling. Although it takes courage, determination, and desire to complete this journey it is not impossible. In fact more and more of us are returning home every year and becoming some of the best residents in a diverse range of medical programs. However, one should not underestimate the pitfalls one can easily fall into along this journey. This book provides insight into exactly what those pitfalls are and how to avoid common mistakes. I would recommend it to anyone considering the non-traditional pathway to becoming a physician.

Keith Morgan BSc (McGill), MD (RUSM)
PGY-1 University of Ottawa Family Medicine

I want to thank our four Canadian graduates for their time and dedication to writing this important guide on how to achieve your dream of becoming a Physician. As trail blazers, these four RUSM graduates have opened many doors for RUSM Canadian students. You are leaders and mentors. This book will help many students as they work towards their dream.

Tom Harkness
Senior Associate Director of Admissions – Canada/International

From the Editors

This book is the creation of four young Canadian doctors who each attended Ross University School of Medicine on the island of Dominica in the Caribbean.

It was there beneath the scorching sun, near banana plantations and mango groves, under the tropic of cancer, that they toiled away in an attempt to fulfill their dreams of one day becoming physicians.

Life was not easy for these four and living in a third-world country was a challenge in itself, not to speak of their efforts studying medicine. At times, it must have felt as though they were trapped in the tortuous nightmare of Sisyphus. This new and unusual world was certainly not for the faint of heart.

Each has a similar story, yet each has travelled a different road. These are their stories; each written firsthand. Their journeys are individual and unique, but also connected. While each doctor has taken a different path, they have all ended up in the same place: bonded together in the sisterhood of tropical medicine. They have all moved on to gain prestigious residencies.

The telling of these stories was conceived when these four doctors shared their Caribbean experiences in the company of *Alexander Keith's and his many friends.* It is this story sharing that has led to the birth of IN THE JUNGLE OF MEDICINE: Journeys through Caribbean Medical School.

Meet these Doctors of the Caribbean:

Dr. Tiffany Bursey (Dr. T) – McMaster University, Hamilton, Ontario (Family Medicine)
Dr. Vanessa Doyle (Dr. V) – University of Ottawa (Neurology)
Dr. Hedieh Ghanbari (Dr. H) – University of Toronto (Family Medicine)
Dr. Raheleh Sarbaziha (Dr. R) – University of Southern California, (Internal Medicine)

About this Book

This book is a window into the journey of studying medicine in the Caribbean. The writing touches on the highs and lows of a medical student's life and offers very personal reflections on these experiences.

The purpose of the appendix section is to assist current students in navigating their way through the maze of exams and applications, which is part of life as an "IMG" (International Medical Graduate) when at times it seems as though the exams and applications will never end.

This is the important stuff that isn't taught in Caribbean medical schools:

PHYSICIANS APPLY/CARMS/MCC/NEXUS/
ELECTIVES/CORES/LORs/ERAS/NRMP
RESUMES/PERSONAL STATEMENTS/LETTER OF
NEED/ECFMG/ROS

It is all here and explained clearly by doctors who have waded through the glue of being labeled an IMG.

The American author Ernest Hemingway called courage "grace under pressure".
You are about to meet four extraordinary people who more than meet this definition.

Chuck Furey – Ottawa, Canada
Carley Desjardins – Toronto, Canada
Editors/04/01/2014

CHAPTER 1

ONE DOOR CLOSES... ANOTHER ONE OPENS

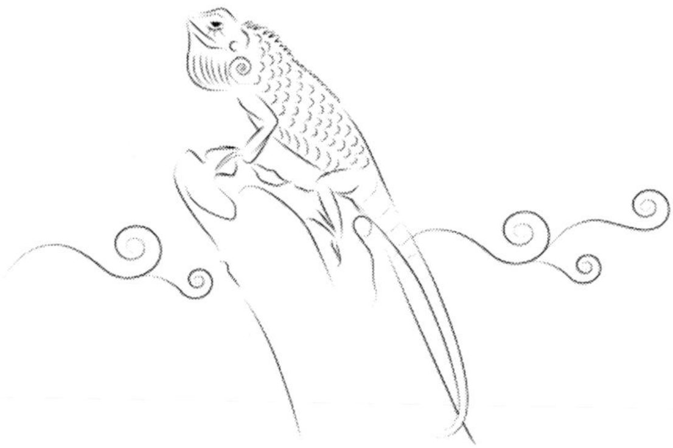

When one door of happiness closes, another opens, but often we look so long at the closed door that we do not see the one that has been opened for us.

–Helen Keller

Dr. T

Molo! That's "Hello" in Xhosa, one of the many languages of South Africa. My name is Tiffany and when I grow up I will be a family doctor! I am thrilled to be able to share my crazy adventure through medical school and residency. Before I get too far, I should tell you a bit about myself. I was born and raised in Vancouver, British Columbia. I went to the University of British Columbia and learned all about cell biology and genetics. I love to snowboard, dive and play sports, especially volleyball.

My first real experience at a hospital was when I was two. I had swallowed a quarter. I did this all by myself and I was so proud. They kept me in the hospital for two days until the quarter finally showed up in my diaper. I'd like to say that I was inspired at that moment to become a doctor after all it takes a special physician to sift through a diaper and find a quarter. More than likely, it was either my mom or a nurse who found the quarter, but the point remains.

Fast forward a couple of decades… I applied for medical school in my fourth year of undergraduate studies hoping that I would be accepted and start medical studies the following September. I knew that the application process was super competitive, but I figured I had a good shot at making the cut, at least for an interview. I felt that I was fairly well rounded; my GPA was good; I had won numerous scholarships and bursaries over the years for scholastic excellence; and I had an abundance of volunteer experience both on campus, in the community and internationally. I was also an executive officer in two different clubs on campus, founder and director of the annual campus softball tournament in which all the proceeds went to the Ronald McDonald House, I volunteered at Vancouver Children's Hospital, was the Director of the Ice Hockey League on Campus and I participated in multiple philanthropy events both on campus and in the community. My most amazing volunteer experience and probably the most heart filled and memorable experience of my life was volunteering in an orphanage in Africa where I cared for over 100 children, many of which were HIV positive. I was also very involved in sports and participated in almost every intramural event and league being awarded Top Athlete of the Year two years in a row. I was a director of a Vancouver Beach volleyball league and also played in many community leagues and tournaments.

But, unfortunately, even with my GPA, extra-curricular and volunteer experience going for me, my biggest weakness was my MCAT score. It was definitely nothing to be proud of. I always hoped that if they would only give me an interview, I could explain why my MCAT score was lacking. I had studied all spring for the exam and about a month before I had to sit for my exam, I lost my very best friend in a car accident. Actually, two of my friends were killed in that accident, but one of them was more than my best friend, she was like a sister to me. I was in the car about 15 minutes before a car ran a red light and killed her. We had gone out dancing and then for a late night coffee; she dropped me off at home, gave me a hug and said "see you tomorrow" and that was the last time I ever saw her again. I was supposed to sleep over at her house that night, but at the last minute,

I asked her to turn around and drop me off because I had to work in the morning. Sometimes I feel guilty for asking her to turn back, thinking that maybe if she hadn't, she would not have been at that intersection at that moment. Other times I think, I too could have died that night. Losing my best friend was devastating. She meant the world to me and I hold onto and cherish her in my heart forever. Between family events, viewings, funerals, community vigils and celebrations of life, I was physically and mentally exhausted. I tried to study between all of the emotion and commitment, but every time I was alone and finally found time to focus, all I could do was cry and think about her. I wondered if I should postpone my test, but I had already registered and paid the fee. In retrospect, I should have probably deferred it and written it in the fall, but my head was just not in it and I know I could have done better. Still, I am stuck with the MCAT scores I had, although not strong, I figured if I could only get a chance at an interview, I could explain.

I didn't even think about applying to other provinces when I applied to medical school. I couldn't afford it. I was on a serious student budget. Each application costs somewhere from $40-150 dollars and I didn't have enough money to spread my applications across the country. In retrospect, it would have been cheaper than going to school in the Caribbean, but the money was just not available at the time. I managed to pay for university on my own with little assistance from my parents. I worked part-time on weeknights and weekends as a lifeguard and swimming instructor, and paid for my housing, groceries, bills, tuition and books with the money I earned. I did it on my own and I was proud of myself for what I had accomplished. But with no extra money to spare, I couldn't afford to apply to med schools across the country.

When I applied to UBC, I thought I had a good chance. I thought that I would at least get an interview. After waiting nervously for the mail each day, my fate was finally delivered and, unfortunately, it was a nicely written rejection letter telling me that I was close, but not close enough. Because my application score fell just short of an interview, they invited me in to talk to one of the medical school academic advisors who would go over my application with me one-on-one and help me in areas I could improve on for the following year. The advisor looked over my application and said that I had a strong application, but it would just take some time before I got in. There are only so many spots, some of which are reserved for out-of-province and international students. The advisor suggested I work on my Master's degree and continue to do volunteer work. I left feeling a bit defeated. It's not that I didn't have enough experience; it was that there were only so many spots and I would have to keep buffing up my application and try again next year.

Some time after, I remember coming out of a biology class one day and seeing this poster hanging on the wall with a doctor in scrubs playing beach volleyball on a gorgeous Caribbean beach. I was sold! I wanted to be a doctor, I loved beach volleyball and I definitely wanted the experience of living in the Caribbean. After doing my research into the various international medical schools, I realized there were tons of schools in the Caribbean, some bigger than others, some more expensive than others, some that were accredited in more places than others, and most importantly, I started to realize that there were many Canadians who had gone abroad for medical school and found their ways back to Canada to practice in all sorts of fields.

After doing my research, I narrowed it down to two schools: Ross University School of Medicine (Dominica) and St. George's University (Grenada). Both on beautiful Caribbean islands, both great medical schools, and both well recognized with graduates all over the USA and Canada. I initially applied to both schools, but later chose to pursue Ross University – partly because tuition was lower, partly because I preferred their semester outline, and mostly because I learned a friend of a friend had gone to Ross and was not only successful in becoming a physician, but loved his entire experience.

To be honest, I had never even heard of Dominica. I initially thought it was the Dominican Republic, but soon learned the difference between Dominica (pronounced Dom-in-ika) and the Dominican Republic. Dominica, it turns out, is one of the most stunning and gorgeous countries in the Caribbean.

After being accepted into Ross University School of Medicine, I had three months to get my life together. I was moving to the Caribbean, starting a new adventure, and a new journey. I was excited and nervous at the same time. I had just started dating someone new and worried that when I left for medical school, I might not ever see him again. We had really hit things off! He was funny, athletic, caring and an all-around sweetheart (not to mention good looking). The more time I spent with him leading up to my departure, the closer we grew together and the more I was falling for him. I had no idea when I said goodbye to him at the airport the day I flew to Dominica that six years later we would be married and the crazy roller-coaster of medical school and residency would all be a blur!

Dr. V

I come from the most easterly part of North America, Newfoundland and Labrador, where perseverance is a part of our collective DNA. You cannot survive on a rock in the mid North Atlantic without stamina and a wonderful sense of humour. Newfoundlanders have lived here for more than 500 years.

I grew up in a small coastal town called New Ferolle, which is located on the North West coast of the island, where my family has owned and operated a fishing business for more than 60 years. It was here as a young girl that I dreamed of being a physician. My mother tells a story of me posting a sign on my bedroom door that read "Vanessa Doyle, MD" when I was just 6 years old. The dream began at a young age for me. My father, of course, tried to steer me toward the business our family had operated for generations.

Through my high school years I found myself drawn to the sciences as empirical evidence meant more to me than the hidden floral messages of poems and short stories. I liked discovering new ideas through science. These interests led me to a Biology degree at St Francis Xavier University located in Antigonish Nova Scotia and to eventually work for a pharmaceutical research company after graduation. This time in my life, while exciting, was still unfulfilling. There existed a void in me that could not be avoided.

I went back to university having been accepted into the fast-track nursing program. This is a program that allows certain students to complete a four-year Bachelor of Nursing degree in two years. Once completed, I worked for a major hospital in the cardiology ward and then later in community health. It was a fascinating time in my life for I had taken my first steps through the doorway of the hallowed halls of medicine.

Having worked as a Cardiology and Community Health nurse for three very productive years, I decided to apply to medical school. I only applied to one medical school in Canada, Memorial University, in my home province. This school accepted 60 new students per year into its medical program and the competition was fierce with thousands applying. In hindsight, I should have applied to other Canadian medical schools as well, but I was naive and had no direction in this regard. I limited my chances considerably. Canada has 17 medical schools and I would advise anyone thinking of applying to go long and wide. In some years, Canadian medical schools receive 14,000 applications for 2,400 positions – yikes!

At any rate, Memorial University did not select me as a successful candidate. To say that I was very disappointed would be an understatement. I carried on nursing and tried my best to keep my spirits up. A few weeks after this rejection, I was visiting my family doctor and he introduced me to his medical student: Michael VanVliet. It was Michael who told me not to give up the dream and to fight on until I achieved it. He was amazing and so positive in his comments to me. Michael was in his 10th semester at Ross University School of Medicine and he encouraged me to apply and start as soon as I could. Michael is now a practicing ER physician in British Columbia and continues to inspire and mentor Canadians from across the country who are attending Ross University School of Medicine.

I applied to RUSM on November 5, 2007 and was accepted into the program one month later on December 5, 2007. I flew to Dominica to begin lectures on January 4, 2008. I was a very happy person: eager, happy, and proud! This was my chance and I was set to earn it.

I should mention that I did look at medical schools in Ireland, Poland and other countries, including elsewhere in the Caribbean, like AUC, Saba and St George's.

Saba was too small and confining for my liking. Although it is a small, but very good program, it appeared to have some limitations. The program at St George's also looked very good, but I didn't like that they took a semester off each year. This to me was wasting time and time was too precious a commodity for me.

Here are the tuition costs for the three schools that I seriously looked into:

AUC
St. Maarten
$16,900 - Basic Science
$18,900 - Clinical

St. George
Grenada
Terms
Term 1&2: $22,414
Term 3&4: $30,660
Clinical - $22,625

Ross
Dominica
$18,825 - Basic Science
$20,775 - Clinical.

You should be aware that all tuition rates in Caribbean schools are paid in US dollars. It is very wise to watch the Canadian dollar closely and to move all or part of your Line of Credit into US dollars when it is most advantageous. Some of my friends were caught paying tuition when the Canadian dollar was 0.77 cents against its US counterpart. Not nice!

So, my research kept leading me back to RUSM. I liked that it was a fast-track program and I wanted to leap right into it and get going.

RUSM has more than 75 affiliated teaching hospitals in the United States and their track record for residencies is outstanding. There are in fact more than 10,000 RUSM doctors working in the USA, Canada and other parts of the world. They are in every state across the US and nearly all provinces of Canada.

RUSM students begin their journey to become physicians on the school's campus in Dominica, located in the West Indies. Students complete a rigorous basic science curriculum, supported by cutting-edge instructional technology, including an anatomy and medical imaging laboratory and a simulation center where students begin to develop clinical skills. Students then complete their medical education by taking core and elective clinical rotations in U.S., Canada, and UK.

My journey was about to begin at a Caribbean medical school, in a foreign land, surrounded by mango trees and iguanas. Through the fog of memory, I could see the small sign on my bedroom door as a young girl: "Vanessa Doyle MD". This was my time!

Dr. H

As a young girl, I grew up surround by medicine. Running around the hospital wards in which both of my parents worked was part of my daily after school ritual. As far back as I can recall, whenever asked what I wanted to be when I grew up, I would promptly and without hesitation reply doctor. It may seem that this was mainly due to a lack of exposure to other fields of work, or that my parents pushed me to follow in their footsteps. I didn't choose medicine for those reasons; I chose medicine because of how you can make a difference in people's lives.

My journey into medicine started by enrolling at McMaster University for a degree in Life Sciences. I was keen, ready and dedicated to achieving my childhood goal. I was determined to do well and get into medical school right after undergraduate studies. Little did I know, how hard that was actually going to be?

As the last child of three, with two older brothers who attended the same university, you can imagine how much advice and wisdom was passed down to me, solicited or otherwise. It wasn't only my brothers, but their friends would give plenty of advice on what courses to take, how to study, what to do, etc. They all had good intensions, looking after their "little sister", but as an individual who likes to try new things, this was a disastrous combination.

In my first year I was busy listening to everyone else instead of finding out what learning approach worked for me. By the time I figured it out, it was too late and my GPA had suffered. By fourth year, the fire and determination inside of me faded. I was confused and not sure if medicine was right for me. I kept telling myself that I would not get into Canadian medical schools with my GPA. Despite being involved in many extracurricular activities, having research and hospital experience, I did not have the GPA to add to the mix for a solid application.

After talking to upper-year students and mentors, I decided to do my Masters instead. I thought that this would make me a stronger applicant. With that in mind, I applied to McGill University for my Masters during my last year of undergraduate studies. All the while, several of my good friends had been accepted to Caribbean medical schools and were leaving. They kept asking me to join them and not bother with my masters. I kept telling myself no, and that with my Masters I should be able to get into a Canadian medical school.

I moved to Montreal, and started my master's program in Dental Science. I worked hard in my graduate courses and published a number of research articles. I attended conferences, being a presenter at a few, hoping that this would strengthen my application. It was that time of the year, I wrote my MCAT and prepared my applications for Canadian medical schools. I thought I would have a good chance as I was doing my Masters at a prestigious school and had publications under my name. My bubble burst when I got my rejection letters in the mail. With those letters in hand, I asked myself, now what? I don't want to continue research as a PhD candidate. How will I become a doctor? How will I do this? I talked to my friends who were studying medicine in the Caribbean and I decided to apply to the

Caribbean schools. My only hesitation was if I would be able to return to Canada to practice. I knew a lot of friends who were completing residencies in the US but I did not want that. I wanted to return to Canada, to be close to family, friends, and for another reason. I was dating someone I really liked and he had been very supportive through this whole process, albeit it was only the beginning of my journey in medicine. I wasn't sure what was going to happen if I were to leave and not come back to Canada.

I spoke with my brother's friend who was doing her residency in Canada after studying in the Caribbean. After talking with her, I knew there was hope and I could achieve my goal. I could even come back to Canada like her and practice. Once again, I had hope and determination. I researched several schools and submitted my applications, my top choice being Ross University for its condensed time on the island and lower tuition – though nothing close to Canadian tuition fees. In December 2006, I received my acceptance letter from Ross University. As I read, "congratulations, you have been accepted", I felt relieved and ecstatic. My dream had come true and I was on my way to becoming a doctor.

Dr. R

Let's start with a bit about me pre med-school. I started my pursuit of higher education at the University of Toronto. I had turned 18 and just moved out on my own. I was excited, but, like most first-year students, mainly oblivious. I remember packing up a box of random things and driving down to campus with my mother. My parents weren't agreeable to me moving out on my own and my father decided not to be part of the move. But I was 18 and, although raised by Iranian parents, I was primarily Canadian and needed to release myself from the tight leash that had been imposed on me.

So, my first two years of undergrad were focused on getting to know myself and the world around me. I learnt basic survival skills, explored downtown Toronto and relished in the idea of going out without a curfew. But all of this soul-searching wasn't without affect on my studies. I was generally missing-in-action with anything related to classes and academics. It wasn't that I didn't want to learn in class, but I was far too busy learning from the new world around me.

The affect on my academic performance was distressing because I knew I wanted to be a physician. By the time my third-year rolled around, I got myself in check and became the same "little miss nerd" that I was in high school. By this point it was too late. Applying for medical school is a rigorous, unforgiving and blind process where grades from all four years are taken into account. I did well in my third and fourth years. In fact, I did so well that my overall GPA was 3.4/4 after being barely a 2.0 in the first two years! With 14 medical schools in Canada and only a handful of them accepting out-of-province students, thousands of applicants (national and international), and many applicants with masters and PhDs, I decided to not apply to medical school during my fourth year of undergrad. I knew that a 3.4 GPA was not enough to even get me an interview.

Instead, I did what I always dreamed of doing: I travel! I ventured out of Thornhill, Ontario (a suburb North of Toronto) and pranced around the world. It was during my globetrotting that more soul-searching occurred and the decision that I needed to get out. Not just move out of my parent's home, but also I needed to leave the country altogether. I decided to apply for my Masters degree. In Canada this is a natural reflex for poor, unwilling biology majors after their dreams of medical school have been crushed. So, I applied all over Europe and Australia.

During this time, the light of medicine was still burning somewhere in my mind. I continued to dream of someday becoming an MD. I knew that as a physician I could help people, travel, have a stable life and explore science. My plans were to finish my Masters Degree and then move on to medicine, but I wasn't sure when or how.

That is when my friend appeared. We first met in Biology 151 in Convocation Hall on U of T campus; a hall that wedged over 1500 students in lecture. A class in "Con Hall" meant a professor that you never met and whose silhouette you could barely make out as he lectured somewhere in the distance. My friend and I would chat about our dreams of travel, medicine and of the constraints U of T had placed on our young souls. I recall stories of my friend's uncle who was a physician in Washington, DC. Far off in America, the land of dreams. And he trained in the Caribbean! He trained medicine in the Caribbean. How was that so?

One day my friend was gone. He disappeared without a trace. It was just me again and "the machine". Downtown Toronto had lost its spunk. I was bored and felt my life was not going in the direction I had hoped it would. It was around this time that I received acceptance to the Masters in Evolutionary Biology program in England and Australia. I was going to move after debating between the beaches of Australia or the sophistication of London. A part of me was excited, but my soul still felt disappointed. And then he reappeared. It turns out, my friend had left us to begin medical school in the Caribbean. When we finally met again, he showed up to my door wearing shorts, a tan and a smile. He didn't even let me consider giving up my dream. "Come to the Caribbean with me Rah," he held out his hand. "We can live our dreams!" And that is how I ended up finally pursuing the one thing I knew I wanted for so long.

CHAPTER 2

A LEAP OF FAITH

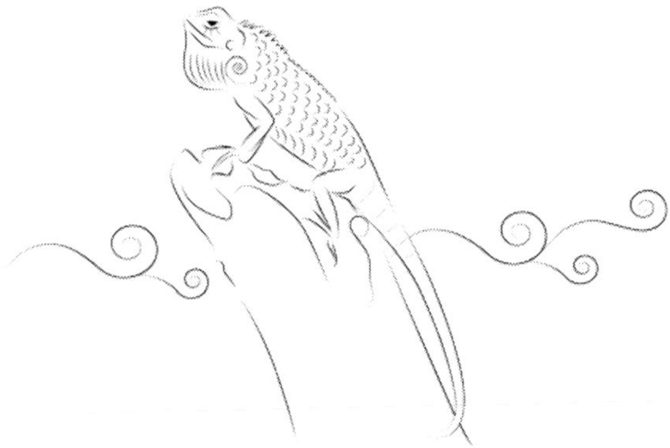

The most difficult thing is the decision to act, the rest is merely tenacity.

–Amelia Earhart

Dr. T

Acceptance letter: check! Now the preparation. I was going to be moving to the Caribbean for a year and a half. Where do you start? I had to break the news to my family, get some serious student loans, book my plane tickets, get my vaccines updated, find an apartment to rent in the Caribbean, shop for both summer and professional clothes, renew my passport, get my school supplies and the list goes on. The only way to get things done was to make a gigantic to-do list.

Knowing that I was moving away for who knows how long was an interesting feeling. I am not sure I can put words to how I felt. Excited for the opportunities and adventures I was about to experience, but at the same time feeling somewhat lost not knowing when I would be back home for good. I knew in my heart that I would be coming back home to Canada to practice medicine eventually, but I also could appreciate the reality and struggles that international medical school graduates face when returning to Canada. I knew I would have to work extremely hard. What I did not know at that time was exactly how exhausting and emotionally draining it would be to fight to get back to Canada.

Packing my apartment was the hardest part. I absolutely loved my apartment; it had been my home throughout university. I was living close to the beach, close to a ton of fun little shops and restaurants. I had so many wonderful memories in that place. I started packing all of my stuff into boxes, keeping everything from my mismatched hand-me-down dishes, to my pencil crayons and Winnie-the-Pooh bed sheets. I figured when I eventually moved back to Canada, I would need all this stuff again not really thinking at the moment that by the time I got back to Canada, I'd likely be a physician and would probably not want or need my old plastic, cracked dish-rack that I purchased at the dollar store. I moved all of my stuff to my parent's garage. I also had to redirect all mail to their address; I didn't realize how many places I needed to change my address – everything from banking to my gas station points card. While I was away in medical school, my dad opened my mail and would send me anything I needed wherever I might be at that time. Thank you, dad!

I could only bring two suitcases and a carry-on with me on the airplane. Seriously, where do you begin when it comes to packing all you might need to live in a foreign country for the next four years in two suitcases?

I had no idea what to expect – would I be able to get my vibrant neon-coloured Post-It Notes in Dominica or did I need to pack a bunch? Yes, this was one of the very important things that ran through my mind. I use Post-its for everything! My friends laugh at me because I have them stuck to everything, but they are seriously vital to my studying!

Guided by my list of everything I might need, I had to make some sacrifices and reassess my "necessities" as my suitcases overflowed. Here's a list of some things you should consider packing if you are moving to the Caribbean for medical school:

- Bathing Suit
- Shorts
- T-Shirts/Tank Tops
- Jeans (Protect yourself from Mosquitoes at night)
- Socks/Undies/Bras/Sports bra
- Gym Clothes
- Dress Clothes for Clinics
- Sweater (Remember your lecture halls/library are all air-conditioned)
- Sweat pants (For studying)
- Towel
- Hat
- Sunglasses
- Short Hip Length White Lab Coat (For Clinic)
- Sandals x2
- Running Shoes
- Professional Dress Shoes
- Laptop
- Cell phone (you can buy a local sim card)
- Phone charger
- Pictures from home of friends and family
- Snorkel Gear
- Photocopy of Passport
- Hair straighter and dryer

Remember most of this stuff you can buy on the island, but if you have your favorite brand, you might also want to bring it with you:

- Bug Spray
- Sun Screen
- Shampoo/Conditioner
- Toothpaste
- Toothbrush
- Razors
- Shaving Cream
- Lotion
- Glasses/Contacts & Contact Solution
- Q-Tips
- Hairbrush

- School supplies (pens, pencils, eraser, binder, paper, post-its etc.)
- Laundry bag
- Tylenol/Advil
- Vitamins

Almost all the apartments come ready with bed linens; dishes, pots and pans; a microwave; internet; and air conditioners waiting for you when you arrive. Every semester, new students arrive and the fourth semester students leave the island. When they leave, often times you can buy used things such as fans, binders, textbooks and all sorts of other things that might interest you.

Where was I going to live? We are very fortunate to have a website put together by the university with all the different housing options in Dominica. I wasn't very picky; I just wanted to be close to campus. There are so many beautiful apartments and depending on what you want to spend and what you are looking for. I found this stunning yellow apartment that seemed to have everything I would need. And so my new address became "The Yellow House at the bottom of the hill in Banana Trail". Seriously, this was actually my new address, and when I came back to the USA for clinical rotations, I listed it as one of my addresses in the past five years at the border.

Telling my family was an interesting experience. Medical school? Few people in my family have gone to university let alone medical school. We don't have any physicians in our family, so there was never any expectation to become a doctor. My parents were always very supportive of anything their children decided to do, so as long as we were happy.

"You are going where for medical school?" Dominica. No one has ever heard of this beautiful magnificent island and every time I said I was moving there, people assumed I meant the Dominican Republic. "Medical school in the Caribbean?" A lot of people had never even heard of medical schools in the Caribbean. Usually, this question was followed by "Why not in Canada?" That's a questions I a lot. Sometimes I felt embarrassed explaining to people that the reason I was leaving was because I did not get into UBC. People seemed to assume that I would get into medical school in Canada. I found that a lot of my friends and family didn't understand why I didn't get in. And it was hard to explain that there were many reasons I didn't get into medical school in Canada. For starters, there are limited spots each year. In British Columbia we only have one medical school for the entire province. The year I applied, there were less than 80 spots available of which some are reserved for out-of-province students and international students. I just didn't make the cut and I was more determined than ever to prove to UBC and Canada that they made a mistake by not accepting me and that I would work harder than ever to get back to Canada.

I got a lot of negative comments from a couple of people telling me what a silly idea it was to spend all of this money to go away for medical school saying that I would "never make it back to Canada". I didn't let it get to me. Most of my friends and family were extremely supportive, but also super sad to see me go. The worst feeling was the thought that I would be so far away from home and unable to help my friends and family when they might need me over the next four years. Life is short and I couldn't help but think about all that I would be missing from weddings to birthdays, celebrations, births and funerals.

Money. How the heck was I going to pay for my education? At the time, I calculated that my tuition would cost me roughly $150,000 for four years and of course that didn't include living expenses. Ouch! I was already in debt from my Bachelor's degree. So, I went to my bank where they offered Professional Lines of Credit for medical students and was pre-approved (without a co-signer) for $170,000. Perfect! I figured that was all I needed. It was enough to pay tuition and would leave me $5,000 a year to live on. I was also eligible for more Canadian (both provincial and national) student loans because Ross University was a recognized school, so I planned on applying for those as well. I was a student and had lived like one for the last four years, so what was another four years of eating Kraft Dinner? If I needed more money, I could always apply for more later. In that moment, all I cared about was having enough money to pay tuition. The rest would sort itself out; there was no need to worry.

By this point, all that was left was quitting my job and saying goodbye to family and friends. The good-bye parties never ended. I made every effort to see everyone before I left and spend as much time with my new partner (then) and now husband!

Dr. V

Getting ready for Dominica was no easy task. I had a husband, a house and a job. I put in my notice at Eastern Health where I worked. I began packing up my house to ready it for rent. And, most importantly, I sought and received the full support of my husband who has been my rock through this entire journey.

And that was just the beginning. Next, I had to file immigration paper work with RUSM for entry into Dominica, pull together all my medical files, get vaccinations, update my passport and deliver all of this within a four-week period to the head office in New Jersey. Life became a blur.

I knew very little about Dominica except what I had Googled: 240 miles of land sitting on top of the Windward Islands with 365 rivers flowing from four volcanic mountains down into villages with 75,000 inhabitants. The climate and local customs in Dominica dictate the style of dress. Temperatures year-round normally range from 75 to 85 degrees during the day, with comfortably cooler evenings and nights. There are two seasons: dry - from December through June - and wet during the remainder of the year. That's all I knew other than the fact that everyone always confused it with the Dominican Republic.

This was going to be an adventure. I thought to myself, "I am taking a leap into the great unknown, but it was in the leaping that I would soon discover so much about myself."

Physically, I was healthier than I had ever been. I ran three miles every day from my house to an area known as Signal Hill where Cabot Tower stands behind the mountain and back home. My dog Kodi was by my side for every run. I loved the smell of the salty air and the beautiful outdoors, while sweating, breathing, and running the edge of the North American continent. There were days I thought I could run forever. Now, life was about to shift in a tectonic way.

Before heading into my adventures in Dominica, I should say a quick word about financing medical school, especially since it is a private medical school where there are no subsidies or grants of any kind. This was foreign territory to me as governments heavily subsidize schooling in Canada and loans are available to Canadian students. At RUSM, the entire cost is to be borne by the student and arranging the $300,000 required is solely the student's responsibility. I say $300,000 because this amount covers tuition, books, exams, travel, food, lodging, etc. I had met with my bank prior to leaving Newfoundland and arranged what was called a Professional Line of Credit, which most banks make available to students who enter professions such as medicine and law. The bank, in this case, the Royal Bank of Canada, was superb. I presented my acceptance letter to Ross University school of Medicine and within 48 hours my line of credit was activated for use. Incidentally, there are two Canadian banks on the island: Scotia-bank and Royal Bank of Canada. There are many other Canadian banks scattered throughout the many other Caribbean islands.

Our route to Dominica was a circuitous one: St John's to Halifax to Boston to San Juan and finally to Dominica. It was December 29, 2007 when we landed in San Juan. And after so many stopovers, of course, American Airlines had lost our bags. After completing paperwork at the airline counter, we headed to our hotel and crashed. We had an early rise and when we arrived at the airport American Airlines promised our bags would be in Dominica when we landed there. We were doubtful.

After visiting the Ross University help desk set up at the San Juan Airport where you could get cold water and answers to your questions, we boarded our final flight to Dominica. The flight to Dominica was an hour and 20 minutes and the landing at Melville airport was something out of Indiana Jones. The plane swerved and banked a hard left down over a canopy of palm trees and then into the jungle onto a single strip of runway. The airport looked like a tiny lonely outpost. But, thankfully, our bags were sitting at the doorway entrance to customs when we deplaned. We had arrived! It was 85 degrees and the heat was intense.

The ride to campus was along a snaking, twisting mountainous road that took a couple of hours to traverse. You drive through a spectacular rainforest that could easily be a painting. Finally, Portsmouth was in sight and the first skeletal view of the university was off in the distance. We were greeted by a fourth semester Ross student who welcomed us to the campus and then it was off to find our apartment, which we had pre-booked. Our home for the next few months would be on Lizard Trail at a house called Coco Mango. We would later move to Dr. Grell's apartments closer to the campus.

The entrance to the university is underwhelming: a gate with a small sign announcing Ross University. For such a beautiful entranceway beyond this gate, lined with magnificent palm trees running towards the Caribbean sea, the entrance itself is screaming for change. It could be so beautiful with a small amount of money and design. There was a fourth semester student who led a small group of us through an orientation. He showed us the campus, talked a little about university life and then left us to our own devices. Once settled, I quickly learned where everything was, had my laptop configured by IT and set about finding the bookstore to grab a few books I needed for the first semester.

I also learned that all IMGs (International Medical Graduates) would eventually have to register with ECFMG (Educational Commission for Foreign Medical Graduates) and become very familiar with this office as they handle all documentation and examinations as you progress through school. They also issue your medical degree.

ECFMG Fast Facts:

Established in 1956
Private, nonprofit organization
Headquartered in Philadelphia, Pennsylvania
ECFMG issued the first Standard ECFMG Certificates in 1958. Since then, it has certified more than 320,000 international medical graduates.

Areas of Expertise:
Evaluating the qualifications of international medical graduates
International medical schools
Physician credentials related to medical education, training, and licensure
Assessing clinical skills
FAIMER, a nonprofit foundation of ECFMG

The charge of ECFMG is expressed in its mission statement:

"The ECFMG promotes quality health care for the public by certifying international medical graduates for entry into U.S. graduate medical education, and by participating in the evaluation and certification of other physicians and health care professionals nationally and internationally. In conjunction with its Foundation for Advancement of International Medical Education and Research (FAIMER), and other partners, it actively seeks opportunities to promote medical education through programmatic and research activities."

You will need an ECFMG certificate to become eligible for residency. To get this certificate you need to complete:

USMLE Step 1
USMLE Step 2 CK
USMLE Step 2 CS

On my first night, I sat on my little balcony with a cold Kubuli firmly in hand, overlooking the Picard River, watching a young iguana slide along a mango tree 15 feet from where I was sitting. I would see him every morning thereafter until I moved apartments the next semester. This little green unassuming creature became my good luck charm.

Tomorrow was orientation and in a few days after, the white coat ceremony.

Surrounded by a canopy of green foliage, frogs chirping back and forth in the marshes and fireflies flitting across the blackened sky, my husband and I witnessed a spectacular shooting star cross the great expanse of the heavens above us. It was a good omen I thought as I turned in for my first of many sleeps under the Tropic of Cancer.

Dr. H

After receiving my acceptance letter for the May 2007 class at Ross University, I was ecstatic and nothing could ruin my mood. I was finally going to follow my dream in becoming a doctor. I felt emotionally ready for my new adventure. My mission was to finish medical school and obtain a residency spot back in Canada. I was so involved in trying to prepare things for my travel and new adventure that I had forgotten that I needed to finish my Masters before leaving. Thanks to my then boyfriend (now husband) I was able to quickly write my thesis and submit for review. With minor adjustments to my thesis, it was ready for final submission. With the Masters out of the way, I could re-focus on my upcoming adventure in the Caribbean.

To ensure that I didn't forget anything for my journey, I made myself a checklist of to do items. This is how I was going to keep myself on track, even to this day I use to do lists everywhere. I remember the thing that made me most nervous was the thought of how was I going to pay for medical school. When I looked at the amount that it would cost by the end, I was scared. We are talking about approximately $160,000, not Canadian, but US dollars. I remember after that I kept a close watch on the US exchange rate. I had saved most of my pay from my part-time job at the local Starbucks, but that was not enough to get me through even one semester at Ross. Feeling terrified about this, I sat down with my parents to try to figure it out. After much talk and sorting of things, we had figured out how I was going to pay for medical school. My parents were great by supporting me for part of my tuition and were also able to co-sign for a professional line of credit. With their help and several of their signatures, I was now the proud owner (technically borrower) of the biggest loan of my life. I also applied for Ontario Student Loans to help with living expenses at school. I thought to myself, please God, help me make it through so I am able to pay back these loans. The financing plan was checked off my list, next up: what is this island going to be like? What will I need to take with me? Where was I going to live? Would it be safe? What type of attire will I need?

This is when I again sought the help of my brother's friend who had attended Ross University. I remember her telling me the names of the trails in Dominica. She said Lizard Trail, Banana Trail and Moo Cow Trail. After hearing these, I thought to myself, "is she serious?" Are those the names of the streets? After laughing with her on the phone, she confirmed that those were the names of the streets where student housing is located. She was a wealth of knowledge for me. She also mentioned that if I liked particular foods (e.g. cereal, cookies, coffee, etc.) that I should bring those with me or have them shipped to the island as they were much more expensive to purchase there. She also advised me to pack sweaters, as the classrooms are super cold. Talking to her made me feel much calmer and a bit more prepared for what I would be facing in the year and a half to follow.

With all that knowledge in hand, I went online and rented a one-bedroom apartment complete with every household items that I would need, including linens, dishes, utensils, appliances, etc. I was going to live in the "Flamboyant Apartment" on Lizard Trail. Yes, you read right, my apartment was called Flamboyant Apartment, given for its bright pink colour.

As the last days to my departure approached, the piles of items that I was collecting to take with me were growing exponentially. I had gathered so many items that I had no clue how I was going to pack into two suitcases and a single carry-on. Luckily for me, I was coming back home a week after arriving on the island in order to attend my brother's wedding. This allowed me to take everything I had piled up in my room to Dominica. My boyfriend also set up a voice-over IP phone for me so that it would be easier for me to keep in touch with everyone at home.

The last thing to do on my list was to discuss with my boyfriend our relationship and how it was going to be. Long distance relationships are hard and I needed to make sure we were both on the same page. A few days before leaving we sat down and I explained the road that lied ahead and the possibility that I may not be able to obtain a residency position in Canada and may have to live in the US. I needed him to be aware of what he was choosing and the obstacles that might lie ahead of us. At the end of our conversation, he could see the worry in my eyes. He hugged and reassured me and said, “I'm in this for the long haul”.

Now that everything had been checked off on my list, I was set, packed, and excited to fly and see the new island that I would call “home” for the next year and a half.

Dr. R

Being born stubborn has its pros and cons. I inherited this trait from my father and I probably wouldn't change it for the world. My stubbornness combined with my sense of adventure transformed my Caribbean experience from something fantastic into a fantastic experience full of suspense.

When preparing to travel down to the Caribbean I wanted to do it all on my own. I deferred the help offered, "pish posh", I thought. “I can do this all on my own. I've been traveling the world since I was born. The Caribbean ain't got nothing on me!” So I booked my own flights, my own routes, on my own time.

I decided to fly direct from Toronto to Antigua with Caribbean Air (an airline that has since been out of commission). All I can remember was that I packed a bunch of binders (which I threw away a few months later), paper (that I never used), a few summer dresses and a rain-parka. On the day of my departure flight, I decked myself out: I put on my tight Seven Jeans, a pink T-shirt from Holt Renfrew, rainbow Lacoste runners, a pearl necklace and, of course, every Persian girl's best friend: mascara. Oh yes! Mama was ready to be one with the Caribbean!

Maybe I should have figured it out when I boarded my flight to Antigua. The random stares from fellow passengers and the majority of people dressed conservative and casual. If I didn't get clue when I boarded, I definitely did when I landed. Welcome to the developing world. It was a crowded flight, but an even more crowded airport. I land and bam the humidity clung my Sevens even closer to my body. My pink T-shirt from Holt's became an undergarment and I quickly stripped off my pearls. My curly hair that I had spent hours straightening was a 'fro.

I was angry and out of place. The chaos at the airport, the slow service (a trend I eventually understand as “Caribbean Time”) was overwhelming. I stood in the heat of the airport with tears in my eyes. “Where am I?” I thought to myself. I had just spent four months living the good life in Miami and was not ready for the developing world.

My tears went unnoticed. I didn't even have a phone to call back home to cry to anyone who would answer. "Suck it up," I muttered to myself. Either you go forward or you turn back. And I NEVER turn back. So I went to the Liat counter, another airline with an attitude, and checked myself and my luggage full of nonsense in. I don't remember much else from my short visit to Antigua that day: my vision was blurred with tears and lots of unanticipated sweat. I boarded my first (but definitely not last) Liat flight and flew across the West Indies. We stopped at two different islands before the plane descended into a scene from Jurassic Park. If Antigua didn't scare the shit out of me, landing in Dominica did. By this point, I looked like a barbarian: mascara smudged, Seven Jeans rolled up, hair curly and full of frizz, and so grumpy, I could barely speak (which I was sure I fit into my new home). If you have been to the international airport in Dominica, you know exactly what I experienced when I landed and, if you haven't, picture a small room, a runway barely large enough to fit a car (forget an airplane), no lights on the runway, and of course a broken sign greeting you to “Melville Hall”. Oh man, why didn't I study harder in undergrad?

Next, I went through customs. “What do you have to declare?" asked the man.

"Binders, papers, mascara, dresses and I think I have made the biggest mistake of my life," I replied.

The customs agent wiped sweat off of his brow, glanced at my passport, the papers I brought with me declaring I was a brand new medical student and ushered me through.

Did he even listen to me? Was anyone going to come and save me from this mess I was in? I cursed myself to hell as I boarded the shuttle from the airport to the medical school campus. Winding through a rural road for one hour would be beautiful if it weren't for the nausea. I learnt the hard way that the best way to prevent nausea on the road was to stare outside the moving vehicle and not in. Two years of island life. How was I going to survive?

Well, obviously I survived. I admit, it actually turned into a great adventure. And although to this day, I am still grateful to my friend from U of T for guiding me to achieve my dream of becoming a doctor. However, his life advice beyond that key piece was horrendous. "Pack only a few shirts and shorts Rah. Don't forget your rain-parka. Live at the student dormitory on campus and do not make friends or socialize."

So my first week on the island was rough. I chose to live in student housing, which consisted of a room with no kitchen, a single military style bed and a shower that housed exotic insects. I arrived during the rainy season at the end of August just inching into September and I remember walking around campus with my rain-parka. Not only were the locals giving me odd stares but at this point the students also thought I was weird. Clearly receiving advice from a guy wasn't going to make the next two years easy. I guess I had to learn it all on my own. I decided to make some friends, throw away the parka, buy an umbrella, and by second semester, I had moved into a cool apartment complex that had a kitchen, bedroom and cute little bathroom.

So my advice to those interested in moving down to the Caribbean for medical school is: If you know someone who went to the school ask their advice (as long as it's a girl), but also bring all of the comforts of home: sweaters, PJs, photos of family/friends, your computer, non-perishable snacks, etc. Find an easy way to keep in touch with family whether it's Skype, Facebook, etc. And remind yourself that you are moving to a different country with different customs, a different pace of life and that it is temporary, so savor every moment.

Preparing financially was another pain in the tush. Thank goodness for my parents and their credit line. We were able to get a line of credit from TD Bank and without it I would not have been able to enter medical school. I lived conservatively relative to other students on the island. I preferred the local foods (more delicious than the bland fast-food chains options) and I was conscious of the money that I spent. I did splurge every so often by traveling to different islands, but it was a way to ensure my sanity given that I lived in one of the least developed islands in the Caribbean.

Living in the tropics is a wonderful experience. Take a day of each week and explore. Go hiking, biking, swimming, learn to scuba, island hop, drink the local rum, eat (and pick) the local fresh fruits and vegetables, work out daily, appreciate the unique flora and fauna that surround you and, most of all, keep yourself focused and determined and don't ever take your eyes off of the prize.

CHAPTER 3

IN THE LAND OF JACK SPARROW

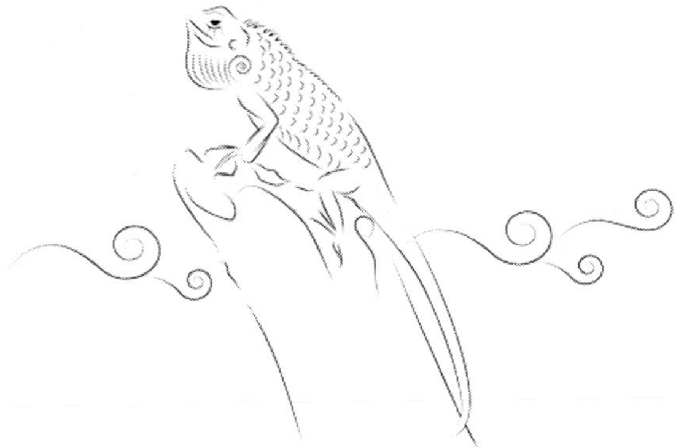

There are moments that define a person's whole life. MOMENTS in which everything they are and everything they may possibly become hinge on a single decision."

— Jonathan Maberry

Dr. T

I hate flying. Let's get that straight from the get go. It took me two days and three planes to get to Dominica. Vancouver to New York to San Juan to Dominica. It was the little plane that flew from San Juan to Dominica that gave me a ride for my money! I remember boarding the tiny little plane with those propeller-like things on each wing and then just as we all take our seats, a man raises his arm and says that there is a leak in the ceiling of the airplane and it was dripping water on his seat. If that didn't freak me out enough, the flight attendant announces that we need to change some people's seats to even out the weight on each side of the plane. I was completely petrified; I kept praying that I make it to the island alive!

It was a beautiful trip over the Caribbean, many different islands, and sparkling blue waters. As we approached Dominica all I saw was this luscious, breathtaking mountainous island covered with palm trees and surrounded by glistening aqua blue water. As the plane started its descent, I was really confused as to where exactly he planned on landing the plane. The plane was flying through the Jungle Mountains and I swear if I could put my hand out the window I'd be able to touch the trees. I thought for sure we were going to catch the wing of the plane on one of the trees and crash somewhere in the middle of those crazy Jungle Mountains. Then, out of nowhere, a runway appears, and I mean out of nowhere! We suddenly make a quick drop – the very quick kind of drop where your entire intestines are up in your throat, worse than an amusement park ride or an elevator out of control. Everyone gasped and the lady next to me grabbed my hand and seconds later we made contact with the ground. We all clapped and cheered truly thankful to be alive. At the end of the runway was a plane that had crashed sometime ago (no one was hurt, but the wreckage was still there). I guess they hadn't had a chance to clean it up yet. Regardless, we had made it! I could hardly wait to see my new home for the next 16 months.

The fresh Caribbean air was refreshing, but hot and very humid. I was lucky my bags all arrived. Not everyone was as fortunate as me. A bus was waiting for us to take us to my new school. We drove around these narrow, meandering mountainous roads up along the coast of the island surrounded by the most magnificent jungle you can imagine. It was absolutely stunning. One of the children on the bus tugged at her dad and said "Daddy this looks like Jurassic Park". A few small towns appeared here and there along the way, but it was hard to see much from the main road. I was so excited. The country was nothing I had ever seen before. It was breathtaking.

We finally arrived at our school and were greeted with a quick tour of campus although I couldn't take my eyes off the Caribbean ocean that existed just meters from the school. I could hardly wait to start exploring! Our campus was just what I had expected. The classrooms were huge with big screen TVs everywhere and everything looked new. The library was small, but seemed to have enough study space and all that I might need from a library. There was a Subway on campus, a bookstore with all sorts of candy, snacks and beverages. There was a beach volleyball court and a large field for sports. And we were introduced to the "Shacks", a strip of several little stands that are rented by the locals who sell everything from fresh-squeezed juice, fruit, sandwiches, chicken, rice, pizza and other delicious local food. I ate there almost everyday. I loved going to the “Shacks” for food because I never had time to cook with all the studying I did. Across the street from campus were a grocery store, pub and Chinese food restaurant. The grocery store was interesting to say the least. It was kind of a one-stop shop that sold everything (like a Wal-Mart, only it was one one-hundredth of the size). Stuff was scattered everywhere in the store, which made finding what you were looking for a serious challenge. We were told to make sure we check expiry dates on everything and if we found something we liked to buy a few of them and not to expect them to ever have it again. Local stuff was very affordable, but imported goods like name-brand cereals was hard to come by and very expensive if you were fortunate enough to find it. I adopted a saying while living in Dominica: “it’s hit or miss”.

I was dropped off at my new house. My new official address would be “The Yellow House at the Bottom of the Hill on Banana Trail, Portsmouth Dominica”. It was perfect. It had everything I would need. I unpacked, hung photos I had brought of family and friends, organized my books and clothes and took a walk around my new neighbourhood. I had lots of large four-legged neighbours. There were stray dogs, goats, and cows roaming in my front yard. At first I was startled by it, but didn’t have much of a choice other than to walk on by them to get out of my yard. There are crabs everywhere! They scurry across the street sideways with their claws up in the air. I saw a few large iguanas; they are so beautiful and are not afraid of people. I would soon learn they would just hang out while you eat your lunch at school. I was told to watch out for the centipedes. Apparently they bite or sting or something and it really hurts. I am sure Dr. V will share her run-in with the Dominican centipede at some point.

Ross University seemed well organized and had lots of activities for new students to do during their first week on the island. We went on several day tours exploring many wonderful places experiencing whale watching, mountain tours, Sulphar Spring tours, city tours and much more. Words cannot describe how magnificent Dominica is. It is one of the best-kept secrets of the Caribbean; so pure, natural and beautiful! Dominica is hands down one of the nicest places I have ever been. I could not wait to do some snorkeling, diving and hiking. I was also excited to start class, but I knew that once school started, I would have to buckle down and focus. As tempting as it would be to lie on the beach and snorkel all day long, I knew that school and studying would come first. At least when I had finished studying or had a break from school, I would have lots to look forward to!

I remember my first day, walking to class passing crabs, cows and goats along the way. I was nervous for some reason, but could hardly wait to get started. Lectures were fairly typical of what I had experienced in undergrad. The professors seemed nice, seemed to care and were enthusiastic. It was a lot of information all at once and very overwhelming. It took me a few weeks to figure out what would work best for me with regards to taking notes, how to study and how to effectively use my time. I sat at the front of the lecture hall, something I have never done before; I was serious about doing well and thought it might make me feel more engaged in the lecture. I took notes and at the end of the day I would hide in the library and review my lecture notes and create my own separate summarized notes that included anything I thought would be important to know from that lecture with the goal that at the end of a semester when it was time to study for an exam, all I would have to do is review my own notes and not have to sort through all the lecture notes again. This method seemed to work well for me. When it came time to study for midterms and finals, I reviewed all my summarized notes and would create yet another even more compressed version of my notes. This was the only thing I would then study for an exam. Everyone struggles with how to study and what works best for them and everyone takes a different amount of time to figure that out. All we can do is hope that we all figure it out sooner than later (and ideally before you make it to medical school).

There you have it: my new school, new home, new life. Next on the agenda was meeting new friends, dealing with the intensity of school and staying sane while successfully fulfilling this crazy dream of practicing medicine.

Dr. V

When I first arrived in Dominica I thought I had fallen into Paradise. The island is so lush and green and beautiful. I saw immediately why scouting film crews selected this extraordinary place for the filming of *Pirates of the Caribbean*. The government calls it "The Nature Isle". There is none of the industrial development and fast-paced tourism clutter that you experience on other Caribbean islands; it truly is in its natural state for the most part. There is an expression in the Caribbean that goes:

"If Columbus arrived back in the Caribbean today, Dominica would be the only island he would recognize".

There is a stark truth to this statement.

Life on the island is slow-paced and easy-going like most other Caribbean islands, and the people are gentle and kind. The country itself is considered a third-world country and the poverty level, at least by North American standards, is very high. Poverty being a relative term, it should be noted that the local people have access to an abundance of fresh fruits and vegetables and a wide variety of fresh fishes from the sea while the sun shines every day.

Unlike the country, the medical program was fast-paced and intense with exams every other week. They have now moved the Foundations of Medicine into an "organs-based program", which wasn't the case when I was there in 2008-2010. The facilities have also greatly improved with newly expanded Anatomy and Neurosciences labs as well as eight new ICM simulation centres. There is also a new library on the drawing board to be constructed next year. Our teachers were, for the most part, very good and were always accessible.

Every day became a familiar routine: rise at 7 a.m., class at 8 a.m., lunch at 12-noon, class again at 1 p.m., study at 4 p.m., dinner at 6 p.m., study again at 8 p.m., bed at 1 a.m. And the cycle continued.

Every ten days or so you have to sit for what's called a mini exam. It is an exam that covers all taught material to that date in time. The exams are always a series of multiple choice questions some with stems that are seven/eight choices long. I must confess it took me a little while to get used to this new culture of learning and testing but in time I fell into the new pattern.

Amidst the class-study-sleep cycle, I met some wonderful people from all over the world who have become life-long friends – a beautiful consequence of studying 4,000 miles from home in the most beautiful of jungles.

When we were on the island, my husband and I started a blog called *Furey of the Caribbean*. We wanted to record some of our memories and thoughts so that we could look back on them some day in the future.

Here is some of what we wrote:

Sunday, July 5, 2009
Of Rains and Sad Dogs

This is the start of the hurricane season and with it the heavy torrential rains. Last night the lightening came and the aftermath of thunder that seemed to shake all of eternity. It was the loudest I have ever heard. The cows and goats roam freely here but last evening there were none to be seen; the weather pushed them deep into the jungle. The rains are not normal rains; they come in heavy thick downpours. It lasts an hour and then the sun. A sun so hot the water evaporates almost immediately. Sometime later the dance of the rain and sun begins again. It is an Eden here where the circle of life and death is palpable and visible at all times.

Dominica is a country full of dogs and they roam wild. Most move in packs of six or seven. They are skinny and scrawny and always hungry looking. You can see the outline of their rib cages; carriers of tropical parasites. They hunt for smaller animals: toads, mountain chickens and on occasion they will encircle a young iguana and kill it; the leader running off with the animal clenched in its jaws while the pack follows. The dogs look like the loneliest creatures from the last corner of creation. Eyes furtive and desperate. Rough and ugly they should be guarding the gates of hell.

Occasionally one is violently rejected from the rest of the pack and has to fend for himself; often scarred and mutilated from a savage fight that ensued.

Yesterday I saw a tough looking dog alone walking the barren streets searching for garbage. His right ear was chewed completely off and his right hindquarter was full of bite marks and sores. A few hours later he lay in the centre of the road dead. From the fight or from a car, a sad black four-legged pile of death. He lay there for a full day until someone finally threw the stiffened carcass into the jungle. Survival here is a daily chore for all living things.

Some medical students are very kind to the dogs. They adopt dogs when they are young; clean them up vaccinate and feed them. It is quite something to see these little strays transformed by the power of touch and the power of love. Dreams of Assisi. These are the ones that will be great doctors, for beyond the scalpels and stethoscopes, the radiographs and the enzymes, they inherently know the secret, terrible beauty of life.

Life in Dominica had begun to settle into a nice rhythm. Beautiful sun, breezy evenings, peace and quiet on an island far away from everything known.

One could only imagine Captain Sparrow standing on the black volcanic beaches of Portsmouth uttering the words:

"It's a fine goal, to be sure. But it seems to me... that a ship like that one, makes this one here seem a bit superfluous, really. "

Dr. H

The day has finally arrived. Today is the day I fly to Dominica. I'm up at the crack of dawn getting ready for my trip. I'm sad and excited at the same time. Sad, because I'm moving away from my family, my partner and my friends. Excited because I'm starting this new chapter of my life. I say goodbye to my parents and head to the airport with my partner. In the car, he is checking over all the things that I need to bring and reminding me of the things I will need to test once on the island.

We arrive at the airport and I walk up to the check-in counter. The woman weighs my bags, tags them and hands me my boarding pass. I think to myself, "This is really happening; I'm really leaving." I grab my carry-on and head toward the security check point with my partner. My carryon (backpack) was so heavy that if someone was to bump me I was sure to fall over. I hug my boyfriend for a long time. I didn't want to let go. I didn't want to say goodbye. Instead, I say, "see you in a week" and continue through security. The idea that I was returning in a week relaxed me. I found my gate and anxiously awaited for the plane to board. I have butterflies in my stomach. At any moment I will be boarding my plane and in several hours I will be landing on an island to start my journey.

After several hours and plane changes, I'm on my last flight. I will never forget our landing. As the pilot announces that we will be landing in several minutes, I turn and look outside my window and all I can see are banana trees and grass. I wonder where is the runway?. The wind was strong and the plane kept on rocking and dipping. It felt like being on a roller coaster. Finally as we move closer to the ground, I see the small runway that we are going to land on. I think seriously, is this it? I close my eyes and hold my seat as the pilot lands the plane. Finally, I made it to the island. We disembark and I'm hit with this warm, humid breeze. I get my luggage and go through customs in the tiny airport. I tell the customs why I'm on the island and grab my bags. Outside the airport, I am greeted by a bus from school that was sent to pick up the newly arrived students. After an hour of driving on a winding road and taking in the beautiful scenery, we arrive in Portsmouth and campus.

I took in everything possible. The island was beautiful. It was rough, rugged and gorgeous. The bus drops me off at my new home "the flamboyant apartment" and I'm greeted by my landlady at the bottom of the stairs. She shows me my apartment and hands me my keys and leaves. As I walk through the apartment, and set up my phone to call home, it hits me. I'm here alone, and this is when I can't hold my tears. I had to remind myself that I came here for a reason, to be a physician and get back home and to suck it up!

I cleaned myself up and walked to campus. When I saw the campus I was blown away. It felt like I was in the United States. There is a huge classroom for each of the semesters, equipped with lots of plasma TVs to show lectures. There is no need to move from one lecture room to the next like when I was doing my undergraduate studies. This time it's the teachers that move between the classrooms. There is a gym, food within minutes of the lecture hall and teachers that are always available for questions. The locals are pleasant and sweet; they are friendly and make you feel welcomed. Everyone lives a more relaxing life compared to North Americans.

During the first few days before school starts, we are oriented to what our semester will be like and were told what to expect. There are tours to the capital city, scenic areas of the island, and lots of getting to know your classmates. This part was especially great: I got to meet classmates, see the beauty of the island and pack my fridge with food. Toward the end of the week we had our white coat ceremony. We all stood and said our oath and were given our white coats. As I was gowned and read my oath, I thought to myself this is it, one step closer to my dream.

Once classes started, we had lecture from 8 a.m. to 5 p.m. every day. The days were long, but they flew by. I would attend tutorial and anatomy review sessions. The remainder of the hours I would hide myself in a classroom to study the day's lectures and review notes. I don't remember where the days went. All I remember and kept telling myself was I needed to do well. There was no room for mistakes.

I enjoyed our teachers on the island. They were very knowledgeable and always available to answer questions. We had teachers that were either flown in from Italy to teach us or ones who had taught in well-known schools in either Canada or the United States. I believe the curriculum at Ross prepared us very well for the USMLE exam as well as the rotations in hospitals.

Dr. R

My first week was the hardest week for me on the island. Nonetheless, I quickly adapted to the situation and learned to appreciate island life for what it was by the second week. My outlook was either I enjoy it for what it is or complain about anything and everything like some of my colleagues. I chose the former and even attempted to blend into the local culture: I went to a local hair parlour and got my hair braided, tanned on the beach, attended my first reggae concert and registered for scuba diving all while preparing for my new career in medicine. The two weeks prior to the initiation of classes are vital to getting acclimatized to island life, meeting fellow classmates and mentally preparing yourself for a very hard path down medicine. Although by the second week I was feeling at home, there were still instances over the next year that confused and even irritated me. For example, there was no Laundromat. Instead, the locals would offer laundry services to the students. Dirty laundry would be picked up and taken to the homes of locals where they washed, folded and returned our laundry the very next day. This was convenient service for us hardworking medical students despite having to sift through random XXL thongs accidentally misplaced in my laundry. After that incident, I learned to hand-wash many of my intimates and nicer clothes. Living on the island was not just about learning medicine for me, it was, in a way, learning to deal with the obstacles life brings to the table and I think I did so gracefully (mainly by ignoring the random thongs in my laundry).

But how were the classes? How were the professors and even fellow students? As a Canadian it was nice because I got to interact with more American students than Canadians. I liked this because I felt like not only was I living in a new country but I was also interacting with new people both outside and inside the classroom. I was intrigued by the different accents, the different parts of America each student came from and the subtle differences in our cultures were interesting to note.

The first week of classes included getting adjusted to the fast, hectic pace of medical school with perpetual worry and anxiety over residency, clinical and crazy co-medical students lurking closely in the background. Our first semester class was located on top of a hill overlooking the lush scenery of mountains. The air was so fresh up there you felt like you just had a lung transplant. And, although surrounded by a tropical paradise, as soon as you stepped into this large classroom (that fit about 300 students) you were immediately transported back to North America. The classes were huge with flat screen TVs all over and the air conditioning ran on full blast. I had envisioned something a little more basic when I considered the state of the classrooms prior to arriving on the island. In my mind, I had a small dusty room, a dinky fan in the corner, an old professor rattling off and a few malnourished medical students in ragged clothing taking notes. Not only was it the opposite of what I had envisioned, but also the classrooms were the most high-tech I had ever seen. Arguably I had attended the best undergraduate school in Canada, but my undergraduate classrooms paled in comparison to the technology at this medical school.

I remember my undergrad professors hurrying off as I chased them with questions after classes, but in medical school, the professors were approachable. I made an appointment to see my physiology professor and he stayed with me for an hour until I understood the concepts taught that week. The professors on their island were either there full-time or part- time. Those part-time spent the rest of their time in the United States or Canada at their respective institutions. Those that taught full-time were usually from medical schools or universities in North America and had decided to either retire or change it up and move down to the Caribbean. Overall, the caliber of the professors was definitely on par with those in North American schools. In fact, they had more time to dedicate to teaching students as a lot of professors in North America have research obligations making them busy and unattainable.

Outside of the high-tech classrooms, the campus itself was quaint small. Small enough that you knew everyone and everyone knew you. Other than sleep, eat, go to class, work out, STUDY and occasionally get wasted on rum, there wasn't much else to do on the island. Once I got into the rhythm, it was great, but initially you feel like the world is ending. "What do you mean there is no movie theatre, no mall, and what ever happened to paved roads?"

Chapter 4

UNDER THE TROPIC OF CANCER

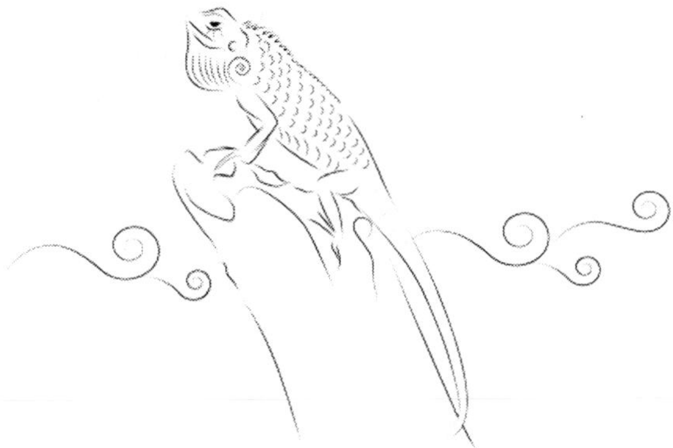

Twenty years from now you will be more disappointed by the things that you didn't do than by the ones you did do, so throw off the bowlines, sail away from safe harbour, catch the trade winds in your sails. Explore, Dream, Discover.

–Mark Twain

Dr. T

To this day, people often say to me, "Oh, medical school in the Caribbean, it must have been nice!" Here is the thing: when I went home at Christmas after spending eight months on the island, I was still my pasty white self; I had no tan. My family was starting to wonder if I was actually in the Caribbean! Well, here are the facts: I was in class eight hours a day and when I wasn't in class, I was locked in a library studying. There was no time for fun in the sun!

Yes, medical school is intense, but you still have to have balance in your life, otherwise you will go crazy. To break up my day, I always found time to go to the gym. I needed that hour to burn some energy and keep my mind healthy. I was also a teaching assistant for anatomy and a tutor. Tutoring helped me keep on top of my information. If you are able to teach it to someone, then that ingrains the information in your brain. Besides, tutoring was fun and a chance to interact with others while learning at the same time. You learn a lot not only from teaching, but also from your students. I tutored several times a week, and although time-consuming, I very much enjoyed it. I also played in the beach volleyball leagues. Our team was the champion one semester! Joining the league was great to get out and play once a week. It was my chance to be outdoors and socialize and take a nice break from studying. I also joined a club called Salybia. This was a wonderful organization that organized health clinics and fundraising events for the indigenous villages in Dominica. I volunteered at one of the clinics and it was such a wonderful experience to give back to the communities of Dominica and also use my medical skills as I was learning them.

So yes, I was an active participant beyond just studying. These extra-curricular activities are essential to making sure you stay sane on the island! You have to have an outlet, whatever that might be for you. I also took Sunday nights off. This was my night to have a nice dinner, watch a movie, Skype with friends and family back home, go swimming or whatever else I wanted to do. After our exams, I always took the next day off and hung out at the beach, went snorkeling or hiking. It was such a nice break to actually enjoy the beautiful island!

I also stayed on my two week breaks between semesters and explored the island. I learned how to dive and became scuba-certified. I did some “island-hoping” and visited other beautiful countries, including Martinique and Guadeloupe. We did a couple sailing trips over to Les Saints. We boated around Dominica, hiked the magnificent jungle trails, went to the hot springs, and shopped in Rousseau (the Country capital). It was always a lot of fun! By having the opportunity to stay during our semester breaks, I was really enjoying the island and it made studying during the semesters easier because I was able to focus on studying knowing that I had seen the island and could do it all again during the next semester break!

I met all sorts of wonderful people and now have lifelong friends from across the USA and Canada. Living together on an island and going through such an intense program really brings people together. You are a gigantic family and everyone really supports each other and does whatever they can to support you. We sat next to each other in class, studied together, celebrated after our exams together and some of us even did day trips with each other. After you leave the island, you may see some of them again throughout rotations in the USA, but many you never see again. Be sure to keep in contact through social media. I think that's why the island is the best part of medical school because you have that support network. After you leave Dominica and start rotations, you are all split up and are usually alone or only with one or two other students you know.

Here is my advice to med-school newbies:

- Don't buy any textbooks until you get to the island and know what you actually need
- Make friends, but not too many – you are there to study! Be cautious when making friends. Befriend the people who are likely to be good study partners. Avoid those that frequent the local bars or watch lots of TV or movies or always on Facebook during class – they clearly don't have their priorities straight.
- Exercise – fit it into your schedule no matter how swamped you feel you are. It is more important to take time to exercise than to do one more chapter of reading that day.
- Eat well – it's easy to eat healthy in Dominica, but it is also easy to choose the unhealthy alternatives, e.g. fried chicken
- Caffeine is your best friend
- Study snacks are essential
- Walk to class – don't take the shuttle (unless it's dark!) because every chance to get some sun and a little exercise is better for your mind
- Sleep – yes, sleep is important. More important than cramming in an extra two pages of notes before an exam. Sleep will keep your brain sharp. You cannot function on no sleep even If it's the night before an exam and you don't feel ready; it is better to get a good night sleep than to stay up and cram, you're unlikely to retain any of it anyway
- Keep a routine
- Take it easy on the night before an exam. Eat a proper dinner, work out, get some fresh air, and get a good sleep. Honestly,

you know what you know and by 6 p.m. the night before an exam, you might as well just relax – anything you try and cram in the night before an exam will likely just be a waste of your time and increase your anxiety

- Make time to keep in touch with your family and friends – they love and miss you and want to make sure you are doing well!
- Delete your Facebook account; it's distracting to studying. Period.
- Use earplugs when you study and bring them to your exams
- Ask for help if you need it and ask early. There are tons of wonderful tutors, tutoring sessions, teaching assistants and professors who are more than happy to help. No question is a dumb question, so don't struggle; get help when you need it.
- Find time to enjoy the island. Hike, snorkel, dive, go boating, visit the market, explore!
- Get to know the locals. They are all so wonderful and have so much to offer and teach you and they are always there to help you when you need it.
- Try all of the fruit – you will miss it when you are gone
- Get involved in at least one extra-curricular activity or club
- Don't worry about rotations or board exams or anything else. Just focus on your first four semesters and doing well – you will have plenty of time to worry about the rest later on!

Dr. V

There's very little wiggle room in medical school with a program that is fast-tracked. And trust me, it is fast tracked: four semesters in 16 months will seem like just one month. A typical day moves at the speed of light. As described by my colleagues, it is true that your time is tightly managed and needs to be used extremely wisely. From the time you wake as you go through your classes, review your notes, attend tutorials and study at the classroom every evening, life becomes a blur. Study, study, study in my case until 2 a.m. every morning. And then the cycle begins again and again and again.

The Caribbean has a rich exotic sound to it from a distance. Going there for medical school is another matter. Your days are so full that even grasping the beauty of the place becomes a chore. I must confess from the outset I didn't take much time for myself on the island as I went there to study. In hindsight, I would have carved out a little more "me time" for sure.

The internet system there was outstanding and Skype kept me close to my family who was 4000 miles away. Thank God for Skype.

The university itself is very high-tech. Internet is high-speed wireless in the classrooms, which are also outfitted with flat-screen TVs everywhere. So all in all Ross University School of Medicine and Dominica provides a very high-tech education.

Most of the apartments are self-contained and also have high-speed Internet. The apartments themselves are acceptable. My one bedroom apartment had a bedroom closet with a couple of drawers, lamps, a nice bathroom off the bedroom with a shower and bathtub, a kitchen area and small living area and cable TV. Make sure you read your lease carefully prior to signing and ask any questions you may have so you know exactly what you are getting into. The majority of landlords are good, decent honest people but like anywhere, there are a few bad apples lurking amongst the good.

When you study at such an intense pace there is little time for leisure. On occasion my husband and I and some friends would go for hikes around the island. There's also a scattering of beautiful private beaches where you can swim and some small boutique hotels that have fabulous restaurants. I'm thinking of the Red Rock Café and also of Pagua Bay Beach and Restaurant Resort near the airport in Marigot. My very favourite was Pagua Bay House run by Alicia and Rick. It is spectacular and the food outstanding. Here is how it's described:

"Located just 10 minutes South of Melville Hall airport, Dominica's newest boutique hotel integrates a simple modern aesthetic with comfortable rusticity in a stylish ocean view retreat overlooking Pagua Bay. With cool Atlantic breezes year round Pagua Bay House offers the perfect place for a quiet get away, where all unnatural noise is replaced by sounds of the surf. Positioned just yards away from the tranquil cove of Pagua Bay where you can choose from a walk on the beach, a swim in the crystal clear Pagua River or have lunch overlooking the Atlantic Ocean at our restaurant Pagua Bay Bar & Grill."

Then, of course, there is the old faithful "The Tomato Bar and Grill" owned by two Canadians: Rob and Whitney. They are super people and the new restaurant is simply amazing. You never forget you are from Canada every time you walk into the place. Eh!
We took a catamaran ride with 50 other students one weekend over to the Saints Islands, which are part of the Island of Guadalupe. It was a fantastic and beautifully sunny day, but the open Caribbean Sea made for some high waves and interesting sailing. While there we loaded up on all kinds of French products: cheese, wine, breads, etc. It was fantastic! The currency is the Euro; so beware of the exchange rate if you decide to visit.

Between semesters you get anywhere from 10 to 14 days off and we used them pretty wisely. On one semester break we flew to San Juan and explored Puerto Rico for a week. Most other semester breaks we flew back home to Newfoundland where we could do some medical, dental and other things that weren't readily accessible to us on the Island of Dominica, including catching up with friends and family. These breaks are quite important because they offer a chance to refuel, regenerate and get ready to start a new semester in a fresh and positive frame of mind.

The islands we visited during our 16 months in Dominica included Puerto Rico, St. Lucia, St. Kitts, Nevis, Barbados, Antigua and Les Saints,

Dr. H

Before starting, I was told of the fast paced, rigorous program Ross offered. This was one of the Caribbean schools with the least amount of time on the island. Knowing this and how hard I needed to work I was ready to buckle down and study. I was on the island to study and make my dream come true and get off the island as quickly as possible. I didn't have much interest in making new friends and being super social. I had made enough friends in university and was very social and that led to me not doing well in my courses. So, my plan on the island was to study and do well on my exams. Little did I know that that was not possible and that I would need friends on the island to get through just about everything.

The first two semesters were tolerable as far as materials and studying went. I liked that you had to understand the process of things rather than pure memorization for the purpose of getting good grades. I remember I would have my condensed notes all around my walls in my apartment and as I was ending my day I would walk around my room and review my notes. This helped me go over my notes. However as the semester materials increased in 3rd and 4th, I couldn't sustain this. I would just go over my notes instead of taping it to the wall. I was also a tutor and anatomy tutor during second semester. This helped me solidify the materials I had learnt by teaching it to students.

After attending lectures, I would study the day's notes and once I had gone through my notes. If I wasn't sure about parts of the material I would attend the many tutorials that were held and ensure that I understood the material. Once studying was done, I would go for a quick workout to burn off the steam and stress. Closer to exams to keep my stress level at a minimum, I would take my notes and stick them in front of the cardio machine, just staring at them while exercising. Not studying or even staring at my notes, especially close to exam time made me super nervous. You may think, I'm crazy for always wanting to have my books close by, but this was my way of coping and keeping stress levels down when it came to exam time. For most, not seeing their books for a while was great, but I wasn't that way.

Through the semesters, I made friends, but I was picky with whom I chose to be friends with. When you are enrolled in a fast past program like Ross, you need to make friends with individuals who have the same set of goals as you. I was not interested in drama, and believe me there was lots of drama and gossip on the island. Whether it was who cheated on whom, who did what, people always had something to gossip about. I didn't have time for distractions or was interested in any of it.

Through semesters three and four, I noticed that my stress levels were climbing and the island was getting to me. I was very close to burning out. I had had enough of it all! This may have been in part due to the fact that I missed my home and my partner terribly. I also found memorization of all the materials that we were learning a bit too much for me to handle. There were times that I would sit in my room and cry. It was looking toward the end product that kept me pushing forward. I wasn't going to give up that easily. I hadn't travelled this far to give up at the first sight of stress and frustration. I relied on my parents and partner for much needed support. I also found it helpful to talk to my friends who were experiencing the same. I continued to exercise as much as I could in order to relieve my stress. Before I knew it, I had completed my fourth semester on the island and was heading back to United States for fifth semester.

You may ask yourself, "Did she do anything other than study?" I tried to find time in between studying to hang out with friends at few restaurants that were close to campus. We would all go out after our exams to the only bar in town and dance the night away. I also did take the time to relax by the beach, dip in the water, site-see and travel to other nearby islands when possible. After exams, I would make sure to take the next day off to relax and recharge.

If I were to do it all again, I would make a few minor tweaks. For instance, I would keep a more consistent exercise schedule and participate in sports. I would also try to see more of the island. I was a bit to focused on my books and whenever the semester was over, I was the next plane home.

What advice do I have for you?

- study hard, but not too hard that you burn yourself out. It is very important to have a life- study balance.
- Try and spend time to enjoy the nature and what the island has to offer when possible. It would have been best if I had a

specific day that I took off each week, maybe that would have been better with dealing with my stress.

- Pick your friends wisely.
- Don't get sucked into the island drama, its not worth it.
- Live on your own if possible and you can afford it. It wasn't good for me when I had roommates in third and fourth semester. It's nice to have your own space and not deal with when your roommates have people over.

Dr. R

Four semesters in the Tropics. It sounds like a dream. Every time I tell someone that I have lived in the Caribbean, I get the jaw-drop, wide-eye, envious stare. And yes it would have been the most glorious 16 months of my life if I hadn't been in medical school, but would I go back and change anything? Probably not. I do realize how lucky I am to have had this opportunity: to live in a new land, meet new people and get to explore all while becoming a doctor. Unheard of right? But the medical program was intense and it was hard (probably harder than being a typical student on the mainland) and I didn't have any of the (simple) luxuries I was raised with. Most importantly, I didn't have my friends or family for comfort and support. Still, the experience helped grow and change me (for the better) as a person.

The program is set up in a rigorous fashion where you literally have to study from the second classes start. You get a two week break in between each semester, which in itself can be stressful enough with all the traveling back and forth to Toronto, reconnecting with friends and family and then having to go back to the island in no time at all. There is also no summer break. Essentially, I finished medical school in three years and six months, which was phenomenal timing, but left little room for vacations, time off, or travel. I did get to island hop here and there, but that was always hurried and lasted only a few days.

I consider myself to have partial ADD, a little OCD, typical female in medicine neurosis and a definite Type A personality. So the intensity of the program was perfect for me. Now if you are a little laid back, used to enjoying life and having little to no paranoia, the intensity might be a little too much for you, but believe me, if you really want it, you can do it (at least that is what I told myself periodically).

Initially, my social life was nonexistent. I was trying hard to focus on medical school and didn't want to be distracted to the same degree that I was in undergrad. Then I remembered this one word of advice my father gave me when I was young and impressionable: he said, "no matter how hard you work, always take one day off to enjoy life".

So early on in medical school, which is where i learnt the real meaning of hard work, was where I also started learning how to compartmentalize life. I would focus hard during class, work out and then go over my daily notes. I would ensure at least half a day off, which turned out to be a very successful method. I would never ever pull "all-nighters" the way I did in undergrad. (I found that studying all night long and not getting any sleep usually led to poor results). I finally learned how to set a pace to my life.

During my days off, I would either go to the beach, eat at a restaurant, lie in bed all day watching TV, or drown myself in my medical school sorrows. As limited as the island is in North American luxuries, there was still a ton of things to do: you could go into town and check out the local markets and shops, take a boat ride, go on a hike, watch the sunset from the pier, gaze at the beautiful stars at night, stand and watch the mountains. It truly was a majestic experience.

I also made some good friends on the island and found the support helpful. With some friends, I would go and study and occasionally joined small study groups. Overall, however, I preferred to study alone. I had a workout buddy and we would teach each other new tricks. I had a friend to go scuba diving with and another groups of friends who I would travel with.

My advice to anyone who goes to a remote place to study is to first focus on the goal. Give yourself one day off each week. In addition to extreme levels of studying, you need to ensure a healthy mental and physical diet, which really shouldn't be hard on the island with all its fresh foods and the accessibility of the campus gym.

My typical day looked like this:

- 7 a.m.: wake up and eat breakfast
- 8 a.m.: class starts
- 12-noon: lunch break. I would eat at the shacks. A lot of students preferred Subway, but I disliked the food and enjoyed the fresh juices and food options at the shacks
- 1 p.m.- 4 p.m.: Class continues
- 4 p.m. - 5 p.m.: Early dinner
- 5 p.m. - 6 p.m.: Gym
- 6 p.m. - 9 p.m.: Study, review daily notes
- 9 p.m. - 10 p.m.: Watch TV or gaze at the stars (I promise you, stars this bright are hard to come by)
- 10 p.m. – 7 a.m.: Sleep

Study Advice:

Create your own study schedule. As I mentioned, I study much better alone. Some people do well in groups. I think most people will find a balance between the two. But figure it out fast, as the program is fast-paced; once you've found your rhythm, stick with it.

Develop a schedule for yourself. Review your notes from class daily and make small cue cards with "high-yield" (i.e. the most important) points and review those before classes. Do you need textbooks and all that jazz? For some classes, yes, but usually the notes given to you by the professor are sufficient. I would wait until you get to the island before purchasing anything. Once you are there you can meet students in higher semesters and ask their advice. Usually they have old texts that they are willing to sell at discounted prices.

And lastly, some words of advice for when you are down and feel like life is too hard on the island:

- No traffic! None. Absolutely zero.
- You are likely to meet the Prime Minister at one point in your time there
- The freshest air ever

- It's peaceful
- Ocean-view no matter where you go
- Possibly your last chance to follow your dream

Chapter 5

AMERICA HERE WE COME

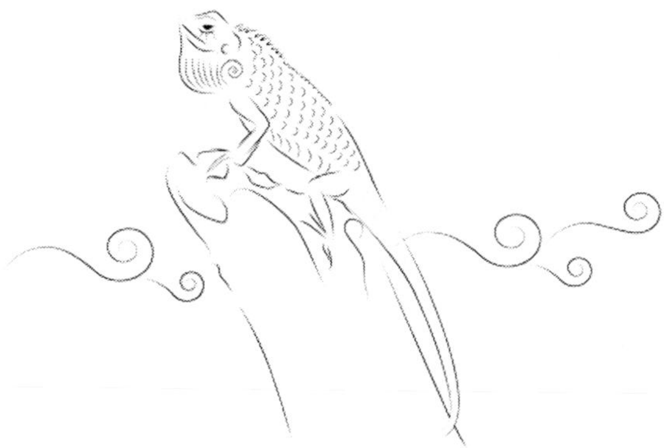

You can never cross the ocean until you have the courage to lose sight of the shore.

–Christopher Columbus

Dr. T

Moving to the USA was a really neat experience. I started off my core rotations in Saginaw, Michigan with six weeks of Family Medicine. From there, I moved to Cleveland, Ohio to do three months of Internal Medicine at one of the Cleveland Clinic inner-city hospitals. Next, I moved back to Saginaw for Surgery, Psychiatry and Obstetrics rotation. Then, I picked up and moved again, this time to Chicago for a rotation in Paediatrics. Aside from a couple of short electives in Michigan, most of my elective rotations were completed across Canada at the University of British Columbia, University of Manitoba, University of Toronto and the University of Western Ontario. So, needless to say, I did a lot of moving around during my clerkship years.

Booking core rotations was fairly simple. I had a few preferences when it came time to picking where I wanted to go: I preferred to stay close to the Ontario/USA border, so that I could go home to visit on weekends; I wanted to live in an affordable city; and, most importantly, I wanted to be doing my rotations at great teaching institutes known for their education. Booking electives in Canada was a bit more of a challenge and very time consuming. Each university has its own application process and so deadlines were important and there was always a lot of administrative paperwork to complete before securing a spot. In the end, however, it all worked out. I have to say, I am very lucky to have done rotations at all the places I did because each rotation was a very unique experience and I would not be the doctor I am today without the experiences that shaped me along the way.

The downside of moving around every few weeks or months is, for starters, just when you figure out your way around a hospital, it is time to move on! Secondly, it can be quite time-consuming securing safe, affordable short-term housing in areas you sometimes know nothing about. I, for the most part, found housing using online resources like Craigslist or Kijiji. As a Canadian citizen, it was challenging at times because you don't have "credit" in the USA, so you could never apply for housing that required credit checks. I guess you could say I lucked out and secured housing for all my rotations at a reasonable cost in a reasonable part of town. Most of the time things like internet and hydro were included. Sometimes my apartments were furnished, sometimes not. I always travelled with my inflatable mattress, linen, night light and basic kitchen needs (two cups, two plates, two bowls, utensils, can opener, small frying pan and a pot). I always seemed to have everything I needed really. When I was in Michigan for eight months straight, I bought a used desk and chair online, so I could study at home (and then sold it when I left), but otherwise I would just study at the local library, hospital or coffee shops. Most importantly, each time I moved to a new city, I had to figure out my way to and from the hospital and grocery stores. Then I had to figure out where the library, gym and coffee shops were and what areas I should avoid.

The first day of a new rotation is always a challenge. You meet all sorts of new people, get completely lost in a new hospital and try and figure out all the politics, protocols, expectations and rules that will allow you to be successful for the next several weeks. Each attending physician is very different; most of the time, they are incredible teachers and mentors and go over and above to make you feel welcome and comfortable, but with each new preceptor, you have to figure out the way they work and like things done. So it's always a bit of trial and error at the beginning. You want to make a great first impression and do things right and that's why I highly recommend always talking about expectations and the "way things work" on your first day. Funny enough, by the time you figure things out and get comfortable at what you are doing, the rotation is over and it is time to move on. This makes you very adaptable! As a student, it is nice because you learn so many different ways of doing things from patient care and management, to hospital protocols, all of which you absorb like a sponge so that one day you can decide which of those ways worked best for you, so you can implement that style into your future practice.

I am grateful that I had the opportunity to practice medicine in different cities, provinces, states and countries. Not only does it expose you to different ways of practicing medicine, but also you meet so many wonderful people along the way and have a greater appreciation for different aspects of medicine and patient care.

Dr. V

I had been to America many times both for vacation and business. Mostly Florida and the Boston areas. I had never been there to live and go to school or work. Moving from a Caribbean island was a shocker indeed.

Crossing the border can be tricky if you are not organized. You need a B1 visa to enter the USA for study purposes. Most times they will allow a six-month entry but in my case they gave me a year. You can go back to the border at any time to renew the B1. The appendix dealing with visas goes into more detail about this. My route took me from Newfoundland to Halifax (where I got my B1) on to Toronto and then Detroit.

I was accepted into the fifth semester ACIM program in Saginaw, Michigan. We would be heading there right after Christmas (Dec 28, 2010 to be exact) flying via Halifax to Toronto to Detroit. From there, we rented a car and drove to Saginaw. I remember it was a snowy, slippery night and it seemed like we drove forever. Then came the lights of Saginaw through a hazy snow.

We rented an apartment at the Green Acres Apartment complex in Saginaw, Michigan. The lady who managed the operations was Jessica Pittman, an outstanding, wonderful resource for Ross University School of Medicine students. She goes above and beyond to make you comfortable, happy and free of worry.

There are many things you need to understand when you move to America, especially the following:

1. Apartment rental and insurance
You will need a deposit, proof of insurance, reference letter. For anyone going to Saginaw, Michigan, Green Acres Apartments, Jessica Pittman is the best: 989-793-4350

2. Driving in America and insurance
Check with your Canadian insurance company and if they don't cover you, call AllState and get covered. You don't want an accident and not have insurance in the USA. Trust me.

3. Banking in America
All Canadian credit cards are accepted and Interac works as well, but if you need a local bank, and it is wise to have one, Chase is the best. Here is a great contact:

Tracy Corbett
1400 N. Center
Saginaw, MI 48638
T. 989-249-5265

Now a few words about 5th AICM and Cores and Electives.

Advanced Introduction to Clinical Medicine (AICM) is a nine-week course for Ross students moving off the island and into the USA. It can be completed in: Miramar, Florida. This course incorporates previously acquired knowledge and skills and augments them to create a bridge to further learning. It is intended to pre[illegible] students for a successful transition to clinical clerkships through additional patient contact in clinical facilities in the United States. Emphasis is placed on improving students' personal proficiency techniques in both physical examination and diagnostic skills. Critical thinking is refined to strengthen the ability to formulate rational clinical hypotheses and differential diagnoses. By the end of the course, students are able to demonstrate improved critical thinking skills and a more thorough knowledge of mechanism of disease processes. There is also an increase in clinical acumen through cogent written and oral presentations in a patient-care setting.

USMLE STEP 1

After completing Advanced Introduction to Clinical Medicine, and prior to beginning your clinical clerkships, you will take Step 1 of the United States Medical Licensing Examination (USMLE). This is a BIG exam because for the first time you are put on a level playing field with all North American students. You NEED TO PERFORM WELL on Step 1. If you hit the mean score or better you are flying high.

Semesters 6 -10

After passing USMLE Step 1, you will be eligible to enter clinical clerkships, in rotation, in specific fields. There are 48 weeks of required clinical core clerkships and 30 weeks of electives.

The required core clerkships are:

- Medicine – 12 weeks
- Obstetrics/Gynaecology – 6 weeks
- Paediatrics – 6 weeks
- Psychiatry – 6 weeks
- Surgery – 12 weeks
- Family Medicine – 6 weeks

The core clerkships in medicine, surgery, paediatrics, family medicine, obstetrics/gynaecology and psychiatry are the basic areas of medical practice in which all physicians must be knowledgeable. They are included in the curriculum of every medical school. Participation in these clerkships also provides Caribbean medical school students with an understanding of the various specializations in medicine.

Electives
The 30 additional weeks are spent in elective clerkships; these must include:

- Eight additional weeks of medicine, which may be spent in general medicine or in medical subspecialties, and four additional weeks of surgery, which may be spent in general surgery or in surgical subspecialties.

USMLE STEP 2
After completing the 48 weeks of required clerkships, you will take the USMLE Step 2 Clinical Skills and Clinical Knowledge. Unlike some US schools of medicine, RUSM requires passage of the USMLE Step 2 for graduation.

I did all my Cores at Saginaw with the exception of Internal Medicine (12 weeks), which I chose to do at Griffin Hospital in Connecticut because it was affiliated with Yale University Medical School. We drove to New Haven, CT and rented an apartment for four months while I completed this core.

Electives come next. Choose them wisely and in areas that interest you. I did three electives in Neurology and went on to match in this field in Canada. Try to get at least two Canadian electives if you are serious about matching back home. Electives in Canada are theoretically available at all medical schools but in the real world and from my own experience here is where you have the best chances; Western, MUN, McMaster, Ottawa, Manitoba, Sask.

Toronto and McMaster are now done by lottery so make sure you get registered for it early.

For those wanting to come back to Canada here is a list of required exams/applications:

- Step1
- Step 2 CK

- Step 2 CS
- MCCEE
- NAC

CARMS APPLICATION

- Residency
- MCCQ1
- MCCQ2
- Licentiate

Stay calm and be patient, it will all unfold over time.

Dr. H

Finally, the time had come, I was going to actually act out and do what I had been reading in my books. I had finished and received the result of my Step 1, and I was ready and eager to get this chapter started. Let's be honest, I was also terrified if I was going to be good at it or know enough material to impress my attending.

Where was I going to go next and when? These were the questions that came to my mind once I had received that glorious notification that I passed the Step 1. One of the many steps in my journey had been checked off – wahoo only a whole bunch more to go!

I knew I had to call Ross administrative right away to get things organized. I knew where I wanted to go and when to start, which was right away. The problem was making sure the rotations had a spot for me. I wanted to be close to home and stay in one place for most of my rotation, as I didn't want to move every six weeks. I had also recently become engaged and wanted to enjoy seeing my partner without the hassle of airports.

After connecting with Ross, I was able to set up two core rotations, one in Miami in Family Medicine and Surgery in Saginaw, Michigan to start with. I was on my way. Only several more rotations to book! I knew I wanted to stay close to home and after spending my fifth semester in Saginaw, I knew I wanted to do most of my cores there as well. Saginaw offered a track program, which I wanted a spot in. This, however, could not be done until later on in the process and there was no guarantee that I was going to be placed in the track.

Still, I was excited. I was going to be in Miami for family medicine in six weeks! The sun, sand and, of course, the hospital thrilled me! Once the excitement wore off, I wondered, where am I going to live? Will I be able to find a nice, safe, affordable place in Miami? How was I going to get around the city? I knew other students had shipped their cars and some roomed with other students. I didn't know anyone and was hesitant to share a place with someone I had never met before. I also wanted and needed to be on budget. I didn't want to add to my loans! I looked online at the available apartments. There were loads of apartments listed, all in different locations of Miami, none of which I had any clue about. Was I going to sign blindly with one of them and send a deposit? That made me feel uneasy, what if it was a scam. After much pondering, I decided that I would go to Miami a bit early and sign after looking at places. I was able to connect with other classmates and discovered that one of my classmates was doing the same rotation and was interested in share rent a car. This helped a lot with staying on budget. Finally, things were coming along and I was going to be able to stick to my budget.

Now that housing and transportation was set, I needed to make sure that I could enter the US without any issues. I knew I needed a visa (B1), but was terrified that I would be held at customs at the airport and miss my place. I had Ross send a letter indicating where and what I was going to be doing and with that I was ready. It's key to be on top of this and ensure that Ross sends the correct form to you. At the airport, I filled out the appropriate forms, paid my fee and, with fingers crossed, waited for my visa to be issued. Once the stamp was placed on my passport and I officially had my B1 visa in hand, I was on my way!

From the experience of finding a place in Miami, I learned that for my other rotations, I had to start looking for a place early. Lucklly, I had been to Saginaw before and knew I wanted to go back to the same placed I lived during the fifth semester. I called the landlady and got myself a one-bedroom apartment for my next rotation: surgery. This was a 12-week rotation in which I learned how to manage trauma patients, learn surgical procedures and manage patients post-surgery. This was an intense rotation, from the early rounds of 5am to late post call days. The attending's can be anywhere from nice to pure mean. After surgery, I was able to complete Obstetrics and Gynaecology and Internal Medicine in Saginaw. I moved to Chicago for my Paediatrics rotation and Baltimore for my Psychiatry rotation.

I believe moving around between cities for my core rotation and electives exposed me to different cultures, patients, and how different health care systems are run. Don't get me wrong; moving around does have its down falls as well. When starting out a rotation, It takes you a while to get to know where things are in the hospital and in the city and by the time you figure it all out, its time to pack up and leave for another place. All this said, I still wouldn't change the experience for anything. I learnt a lot about people and myself. One advice: Try to be flexible and things will fall into place.

Dr. R

So here I was: the Canuck on a mission. I just survived 16 months on "the rock" and now it was time to decide my next two years as a medical student. Where should I do my fifth semester? Where should I do rotations and how do I secure the perfect residency? Although I wasn't quite sure of my next physical move, I have always had an idea of what I wanted and in which setting I learned best. I decided the stay on the island for fifth semester. It made the most sense for me at that point in my life from a financial, social and personal perspective. I had made a great group of friends on "the rock" and we all decided to stick together for the fifth semester. Living on the island for the fifth semester was also considerably cheaper than moving to Miami, and I knew if I went to Miami, I would be distracted by all that Miami has to offer. Staying on the island for the fifth semester turned out to be a wonderful way for me to become better acquainted with a smaller group of students, to explore the island a bit more and focus on my studies.

After passing the comprehensive exam (on my first try!), I knew it was time to buckle down and study. I wanted to be well prepared for Step 1. So I moved back to Toronto, but steered clear of my parents' home. As wonderful as my family is, I knew I had to find a quiet and peaceful place to study. So I moved one block over to my aunt's house. I would study there daily. It was a great experience and I got fed in unlimited supplies of homemade Persian food. I was in heaven (studying aside). I prepared myself for an entire month in my aunt's apartment: studying, eating, sleeping, and, of course, working out. I cannot imagine having a balanced study schedule without the gym.

After I got my Step 1 score in the mail, I immediately contacted Ross and told them the good news: I was ready to move back across the border and continue my path as a medical student. Ross initially gave me a list for all my clinical cores, but I called my friend (again) and asked him his advice: where should I do rotations? How do I move? How do I space them apart? How do I move to the States? How do I find housing? Once again, he couldn't answer these questions the way I would have needed them answered; but, then again, I am a girl and he is a boy; I am an internist and he a surgeon. We are so different! But, let's give the guy some credit; he definitely guided me in the right direction. He recommended that I call Ross back and ask to do my first rotation at a private Yale-affiliated hospital in Connecticut. I trusted his opinion and Yale-affiliated sounded super fancy. Except, I didn't realize that Connecticut is apparently colder than Toronto and that the town had a population of roughly 12,000, the majority of which who are retired. So I packed my mother's M-class with randomness (I definitely had mastered the art of packing by this point, no binders and parkas for me) and my brother and I set on a road trip to Connecticut. We drove from Toronto through upstate New York late in the fall of 2008. Listening to the radio, MP3s, and chatting about the possibilities ahead, including where I was going to live. I had found a place on Craigslist, but the entire car ride down I couldn't get the landlord to answer his phone. I was nervous, my brother seemed indifferent and I don't really think my parents had any clue where I was. I remember about an hour prior to our silent arrival into Derby, CT, the landlord's wife finally called me back and asked me to meet her at the house. It was dark by the time we arrived and my brother wanted to buy some Blue Moon Beer prior to returning to Canada. Except, there were restrictions on selling beer after a certain hour in this town. Really? I was already confused. Finally I met my landlady. A chubby, middle-aged Caucasian female who drove a minivan. She handed me the keys to an old Victorian home. I was going to live with two other girls. One was a medical student from India and the other a 21-year old searching for a husband. I got the last of the three bedrooms, which also housed the heater, so every time we turned the heat on at night I would suffocate as if in a sauna. This room also came with the makeshift bathroom located across the hall. It used to be a sunroom or something. All I knew was that there was no heat – at all. So in the dead of small town Connecticut winter, I would wake at 5 a.m. and leave my sauna to stagger over to the icebox to wash my face and brush my teeth. Showers were only taken at night and eventually I convinced the landlord to buy a space heater for the bathroom (although he would have his daughter come over to investigate the exact amount of heat used weekly). I was miserable; my Indian roommate was homesick and we suffered multiple cultural differences; meanwhile, the 21-year old roommate was focused on husband hunting. We were three completely different girls living under one roof while the landlord's daughter and her lesbian lover were upstairs. I would have to walk about 30-40 minutes in the freezing cold to buy groceries. The walk to the store was tolerable, but imagine the uphill walk back with a bag full of instant noodles and cheap pasta sauce. At least the hospital was close. Maybe a 5-minute walk. I would walk there daily with my layers of clothes and arrive in a quaint lobby where there was usually someone playing the piano. Yes, it was beautiful and helped the thawing process. This was my first real experience in an American hospital setting. At this point, I didn't know the difference between public or county hospitals and private ones. But now I know that as a patient, I am sure that I would prefer a private hospital, but as a student/resident, a county hospital is definitely the way to go for learning. Although everyone is different I think it has been universally accepted in the medical community that if you train in a county system you will leave being able to handle anything. It would be difficult for Canadians with a universal healthcare system to fathom the drastic differences between the county and private systems that exist in the US. Here's a sense of the drastic contrast of the two systems:

County	Private
Patients almost never speak English and are generally marginalized and impoverished	Patients are usually educated and speak English
Nurses don't usually speak English and rarely care	Excellent nursing
Many patients appear after years of not seeing a physician. At this point, they have multiple diseases and all have manifested physically and they usually don't listen to a word you say as their doctor	Patients know a lot about their health and work with the physician to show progression in their health
Patients can be physically and verbally abusive	Patients can be “know-it-alls” and high maintenance
You are really helping those in need	Ok fine, you are helping those in need

You will see everything!	BORING. I am so over osteoporosis
You have to fight for your patients, their rights, your own rights and your sanity	Orders, procedures, imaging studies all get done in a timely fashion

Oh my! Have I convinced you to not work at a county hospital? I hope not. Because despite all of the differences between the systems, I would choose a county system over a private system a million times over. The pathology, the patients, the chaos, I am certain can only make me a better physician and this is where the saying "if it doesn't kill you, it only makes you stronger" comes in.

Overall, the Yale -affiliated hospital was a decent experience. I got to walk through the Yale campus (which was quite similar to U of T campus), and I met some wonderful attendings, residents, co-medical students and patients. Ultimately, I knew that I wanted to see and do all of the things that you read about in the pathology textbooks, and after spending two years on a tropical island, I also knew that warm weather was where I needed to be.

Let's see... I conquered Miami, did the Caribbean, so, naturally, California was next on my list of places to live and flourish. So, I applied to work in a hospital in California. Ahh I was excited to explore the beaches, meet celebrities, shop 'til i dropped, eat Mexican food, and claim my throne as the new California girl. Then I arrived at my destination: Bakersfield, California. Bakersfield made Derby, CT look like the south of France with its level of sophistication. Oh man, was this really California? Smack in the middle of the desert: a city with the highest rate of high school dropouts, highest crime-rate per capita, no one spoke English, meth was more readily available than Kit-Kat bars, and beat up, burnt out gang bangers from East LA had trickled up to the ghettos of Bakersfield (where the rent was cheaper and away from the chaos of the city). Where was George Clooney to assist me with all my medical questions? Damn you Hollywood for lying to vulnerable youth like me!

Yes it took a while to become adjusted to this drastic change from East to West Coast, but it was in Bakersfield where I learned some of the most important life lessons that have helped me through medical school, residency and life itself:

1. Life is not fair
2. I need to learn Spanish and I need to learn it now
3. Alcohol is man's best and worst friend.

I had a friend living in Bakersfield. A cool guy I knew from medical school who let me crash with him until I found a place to rent in a gated community (which us Canadians don't know much about, but is essential when you live almost anywhere in America). I remember walking into the hospital and thinking "Am I in California or back in Dominica?" The hospital in Bakersfield was worse than the hospital in Dominica. Let me give that little island some credit. This place was falling apart from the inside out. The rooms were gross and occupied up to four patients at a time, I saw cockroaches scurrying across the wards, the nurses ignored everyone (including the patients), the patients ignored everyone (including the doctors), but all of this was irrelevant given the education that I was receiving. Within my first week, I think I learned more by touching, seeing and observing than I did in the entire three months at the posh hospital in Connecticut. I eventually finished all my cores in Bakersfield, California and was grateful for every minute I had in this desert town.

Electives are a different beast in and of themselves and it is prudent that you plan ahead. I spent a good portion of my third year looking for elective options in different hospital and cities where I would be potentially interested in the programs. It is recommended that all fourth year medical students travel to other hospitals to expose themselves to programs of interest. I was able to arrange electives at LA County University of Southern California (USC), Cottage Hospital in Santa Barbara, Cleveland Clinic in Fort Lauderdale and Nassau in New York. I did quite a bit of research on the different hospitals and locations that I was interested in, calculated my finances, estimated my timing and set myself on a path of finding the right hospital for me.

Most of the hospitals I chose (with the exception of the Cleveland Clinic) were county hospitals. I immediately fell in love with County Hospital and USC, in particular, and I made it my goal to obtain my residency there. There were many similarities between Kern and LA County USC, so I felt comfortable when I interviewed. During my interview trail, I remember an attending made an excellent point: always go with your gut when you rank residency programs, and my gut said USC. So I ranked and eventually obtained residency and started working at USC.

Although it is a little harder for Canadians to move around the States, adapt to the subtle cultural differences and eventually obtain residency in an American Hospital, many Canadians do it successfully each year. The only holding factor is the VISA issues, which really isn't an issue, but rather a load of paperwork that needs to be completed appropriately and on time.

I am happy that I was able to travel from the East to West Coasts in pursuit of my education. I strongly believe that experiencing other hospitals allows you to meet different attendings, appreciate different styles of medicine, be exposed to diseases that are localized to certain areas (for example, sickle cell in Dominica, Lyme disease in Connecticut and coccidiomycosis in Bakersfield). You also get to travel, make new friends and you will have a good understanding of what you want (or don't want) your educational journey to be.

Chapter 6

IN THE BOSSOM OF MEDICINE

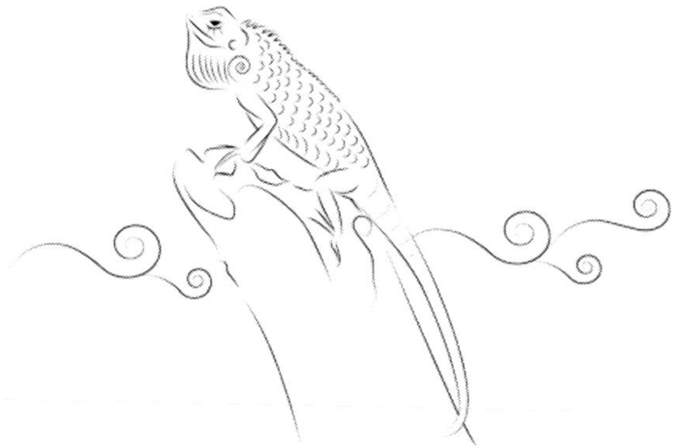

If you hear a voice within you say "you cannot paint," then by all means paint and that voice will be silenced.

–Vincent Van Gogh

Dr. T

Core rotations are just that – core rotation! You have to do them, even if they are of no interest to you what so ever. Fortunately, I am a family physician so they are all relevant to family medicine. As a family doctor, I see it all! After all, we are the front line gatekeepers to pretty much everything in Canada.

Internal medicine is a longer rotation: 12 weeks to be exact. I feel that it is a very important rotation because you get a flavour for medicine in general. I completed my internal medicine in an inner city hospital in Cleveland. What a fabulous experience. You see a wide variety of interesting cases related to all body systems and organs, and you really get to use the basic clinical knowledge that you have been practicing up until that point. It's a great first rotation to start off with as each patient you experience provides an opportunity to read about a different topic when you get home. Call it nerdy if you want, but if you read about the patients you take care of, you will never forget them.

The material also makes far more sense once you have actually seen it in real life. I feel like I experienced it all – from complex, late stage disease processes to rare presentations of uncommon diseases!

The surgery rotation was hell. Well at least that's how I imagined it! Surgery presents a grueling 12-week rotation complete with long hours, stress, no sleep, slavery, under-appreciation, scut work, and no social life let alone time to eat or exercise. Nonetheless, it was fabulous learning experience and I wouldn't have traded it for any other.

The surgery rotation started at four or five in the morning each day with pre-rounding on all the hospital patients before my senior resident arrived at the hospital to review them with me at six. Then, at around eight, the staff physician would arrive and we would do rounds together on all of the surgery patients under our team. Next, we would head to the operating room for multiple back-to-back cases that could last anywhere from 30 minutes to eight hours each. At around six p.m., we would finish up and head home for the night unless, of course, it was your lucky day to be on-call. On-call days seemed to last forever! We would be up all night covering all surgery patients in the hospital, as well as any new admissions to hospital and trauma patients in the emergency room. It was never a dull night. From gunshot wounds requiring urgent laparotomies to patients needing emergency resuscitation. I don't think I slept more than an hour on any shift. Granola bars were my best friend that rotation. I had at least four bars in my pockets at any one time and would inhale them whenever there was a chance. We usually at breakfast as a team before rounds in the morning; this was by far my favourite part of the day. It was a lot of work, but like I said, good learning. There was limited time for studying during this rotation, but the on-the-job experience was rich enough, and with all the questions the senior residents and staff physicians would "pimp" you with all day long, you had to stay on the ball and up to speed with your clinical knowledge.

Psychiatry, in contrast, was a nice break. Mental illness is definitely fascinating and a whole world in and of itself. The hours were great and I was fortunate enough to have both inpatient and outpatient clinic experience during this rotation. I will never forget some of the amazing patients I met and realized how debilitating mental illness can be. It breaks my heart knowing just how misunderstood mental illness is along with all of the stigmas that society has attached to it. I was truly privileged to be a part of those patients' care at a point in their lives when they were so incredibly fragile.

Paediatrics, on the other hand, is an opportunity to learn as much as you can about children. Generally speaking, children are healthy and you don't see them when you do your surgery, psychiatry, internal medicine or even your family medicine rotations. You see them occasionally for well-child check-ups during your family medicine rotation; but, quite frankly, it's few and far between. Try to ensure that your paediatric rotation has some in-hospital and clinic component to it; this will offer a good variety of exposure, and, unless you are going into family medicine, or paediatrics, you might never see children.

Obstetrics and Gynaecology is another wonderful rotation, and like paediatrics, a very important rotation because unless you plan on doing family medicine or obstetrics, it's very unlikely that you will ever get a chance to deliver a baby again. I recall crying when I delivered my first baby; I couldn't help it. It is such an incredible experience to be a part of bringing a new life into the world, and, most of the time, everyone is happy and healthy! No matter what specialty you go into in life, you will always come across pregnant woman. It is important to have an understanding of obstetrics because it will likely complicate your diagnostic and management plan. This was by far my favourite rotation to the point that I contemplated doing obstetrics and gynaecology for the rest of my life, except I wasn't much interested in the gynaecological surgery aspect. Don't get me wrong, I liked it, but I was more interested in the obstetrics and this is why Family Medicine is the right choice for me: I get to deliver babies and then follow mom and baby after the deliver!

Family medicine was a nice consolidation of everything you have learned. I, unfortunately, did my family medicine rotation near the beginning of my core rotations. If I could do it again, I would definitely make this my last rotation. It gives you an opportunity to practice everything you have learned during your other specialty rotations. It is an opportunity to work on your patient-centred approach, clinical exams and physician-patient relationships. Depending on where you do your family medicine rotations, try and rotate at a clinic that does its own obstetrics, inpatient hospital care and maybe even some emergency medicine shifts. I think this additional exposure will allow you to truly experience what most Canadian physicians do outside of urban centres.

Well, there you have it: a sneak-peak into my core rotations. I hope I didn't scare you too much! Remember, core rotations are just the starting blocks; they give you brief exposure to different specialties, which allows you to then mould your electives to your specific interests or in areas you think you would like more exposure. I think if I were to add one "core" rotation, I would include Emergency Medicine. You might get exposure to the E.R. through internal medicine, surgery or on family medicine, but I think it's important for all medical students to be exposed to resuscitating sick patients as well as first presentations of disease, and practicing formulating a differential diagnosis, as well as an investigation and management plan. If you do not get a chance to do time in the Emergency Room, then I would highly suggest doing an elective there; no matter what area you plan on going into.

Dr. V

The first time I heard the words Dr Doyle it felt both strange and exhilarating. Strange because I had finally "arrived" and exhilarating because responsibility had now entered the equation in a very real way. It was time to really focus now. I was reminded of the British poet's words: "nothing focuses the mind more than the knowledge that one is to be hanged in a fortnight" (S Johnson) I wasn't to be hanged, but I was about to undertake an enormous responsibility.

My first core rotation was Surgery and I strongly advise against beginning your cores with Surgery. It is the most difficult core for a number of reasons and should be saved for late in the core cycle. Firstly, you are dealing with surgeons who we jokingly like to say suffer from the " God-complex phenomenon "; some surgeons can be truly difficult to deal with and navigating around their incredible egos can be breathtaking at times. I know this is a generalization but ask any medical student and they will nod their heads in agreement. Humility and surgery have rarely encountered each other. It's just a fact of medical life. This rotation is time consuming but can be a great learning-experience if you go at it in an earnest way. The ego issues are minor obstacles to deal with on your pathway forward but necessary evils to bring you in tune with the real world. Working with a good surgeon can be really quite spectacular and working with a poor one can be distressing. I have witnessed both.

My next core rotation was Psychiatry. I thoroughly enjoyed this rotation. The doctors were great teachers/mentors. We worked at a psychiatric unit in the city and were exposed to many varieties of illnesses. We also spent time at a juvenile prison for young woman. As you know many track programs require students to complete the NRMB board exams after each rotation. I was happy with this because it forced you to focus and it was great preparation for the Steps. During my Psych rotation we were each asked to make a presentation on various subjects. I chose to turn my own presentation into a game of Jeopardy so that it could be both informative and fun.

The other cores were pretty standard. During this time, I left Michigan for three months and drove to New Haven, CT so I could do IM at Griffin Hospital, which is affiliated with Yale University. This was a very fine experience as the teachers were superb and the overall experience very rewarding. I had been approached to do IM there as a residency if I had wanted, but Canada beckoned and it was my sincere dream to come home. This was at a time when pre-offers were available in the US, but have since been discontinued for the most part.

My cores looked like this:

Surgery: Synergy
Psychiatry: Synergy
Obgyn: Synergy
Peads: Synergy
IM: Griffin/Yale
FM: Regina

Of course, cores whiz by in a very fast manner. The thing about cores is to remember to always show up on time be professional, look interested, ask questions and always be the last one to leave. The very last!

Dr. H

The first rotation that I had was family medicine in Miami. Yes, beautiful Miami in the summer time. This rotation was very relaxed and it was what you made of it. You could learn as little or as much as you wanted. We didn't do as much outpatient clinic like you typically expected of your family medicine rotation. We would round on nursing home patients, and occasionally tag along with specialist who came to do visits. I would finish seeing and writing notes on my patients by noon and then I would figure out what I could do to learn more. I really didn't want my experience to go to waste and wanted to make sure I got the most of my rotation. We had several teachers who were very excited and dedicated to teaching. I will also never forget the orthopaedic surgeons who use to have clinics at the nursing home. He was intimidating but a great teacher. I learned how to read x-ray, assess wounds and was even able to shadow him in the OR. I also tagged along with a gastroenterologist what would see patients on the wards. I was able to manage common gastrointestinal problems and change gastric feeding tubes.

Overall, the best core rotation experience that I had was in Saginaw, Michigan. I completed my obstetrics and gynaecology, internal medicine and surgery in Saginaw. The program was very well organized. They had great teachers and the ratio of student to physician was low. My surgical rotation was fabulous especially by comparison to stories I would hear from students who did their surgical rotations in New York. There were two to three students per team, with minimal scut work being passed off to the medical students. You received great teaching from the staff who were actually interested in teaching. The best part of this rotation was that out of the 12 weeks of surgery you had four weeks of trauma surgery and another four weeks emergency medicine. The hospital that we rounded at in Michigan was a Level 1 Trauma Center, which revealed a lot of interesting cases -- from gunshot wounds to people falling off of balconies or ladders. The hours of this rotation were not as wonderful as my family medicine rotation. We would typically start rounding at 4-5am depending on how many patients needed to be seen, and then round with the seniors and staff after. Once the rounds were done, we would head to the OR for cases that were booked. This rotation was the first rotation to be on call overnight. Overnight calls were unpredictable; if you were lucky you were able to sleep for a few hours. However, these were the best calls, filled with lots of adrenaline. Whether was answering a trauma call, doing emergency surgery, there was never a dull moment.

Internal medicine was a 12-week rotation which I did in Saginaw. It was a great rotation filled with lots of teaching and learning. We had a wonderful teaching by the name of Dr. Lambert; he was a wealth of knowledge. He would do our weekly teaching and whatever he taught us was gold. I learnt so much in this rotation and used my notes even to this date to review from.

As for my last two rotations, paediatrics and psychiatry, they were less than ideal rotations. My paediatrics rotation was in Chicago. In Chicago, Ross University has access to two sites for paediatrics. This was the lesser of the two evils. The rotation was "ok" with regards to exposure to common illness in children; however, it could have been much better organized. The exam at the end of the rotation was not an NRMP exam, but something they had put together. So you didn't really need to study very hard. With that being said, I didn't mind that the rotation was more relaxed because I was taking my Step 2 CK exam during this rotation and it allowed me to study more for the exam and more time to see the city as well.

My final core rotation was psychiatry in Gainesville, FL. We were to rotate with a psychiatrist at a psych facility. This was one of the rotations that Ross provided housing for its rotating students. It was about time, after all the money I was putting toward housing, exams and moving around to not have to worry about housing for a rotation was a blessing. This rotation was more relaxed than any of my other rotations. We would go to the ward in the morning and either observe court cases or interviews performed by staff. We dealt with extreme cases of psych and not what you would see on a daily bases in your clinic. Again I didn't mind having a more relaxed rotation. I took the opportunity to read and learn on my own and prep for my next set of exams, the Step 2CS and Canadian exam, which would take place in eight weeks.

Overall, I liked my core rotations, and to be honest you just have to finish your cores. I'm glad that I didn't take more than two relaxed-rotations as I would not have prepared me for my exam and I would not have done as well.

Dr. R

I have already mentioned my trials and tribulations of finding rotations, entering and exiting the United States. Now, I will go more in depth on my core rotations, how I found them, how to excel, what to accept, what to give and what to avoid!

The core rotations - as you may already know - include internal medicine, surgery, family medicine, paediatrics, OB+GYN and psychiatry (some medical schools have additional rotations that they also consider cores). All very important and all required for every medical student in North America to complete prior to finishing medical school. I decided to start with internal medicine and I think that is a great idea for the majority of students. The core component in the majority of standardized tests is internal medicine and starting with this rotation will give you the upper hand especially when preparing for exams and going through your other rotations. It is important to keep in touch with co-medical students, but sometimes it is more important to keep in touch with those a few semesters ahead of you. Doing so will allow you to get advice regarding future rotations, housing options and how to best survive your last two years as a Canadian doing core rotations in the United States.

I armed myself with a ton of knowledge of the better hospitals, the most ideal locations (for me), and then set forth in starting my rotations. When I started my rotations I had no clue "what I wanted to do when I grew up". Some of my co-medical students knew right away that they wanted surgery or paediatrics, but I was as clueless as they come. Maybe this worked in my favour or maybe it didn't, but all I know is that I am happy where I am right now and probably wouldn't change a thing in my windy path of becoming an MD. Bottom line is I chose my path and you have the right to do so too whether it is staying in one city or moving around to different parts of the United States. It really is possible to do your cores in a setting that you consider ideal. So as I began my rotations, I wasn't quite sure the best way to go around succeeding as a medical student. Thankfully, in retrospect, I now know how to maximize my time and succeed in rotations while at the same time savouring the minimal free time you do have.

Starting the first rotation can be scary. First time in a hospital. First time around patients. Wondering “what is that smell?” Why the heck are residents so cranky? Who are these weird attending who keep asking you questions in front of a small audience? What do you mean you have to run in front of the team rounding and gather the charts? I'm sorry I have to pay for this hospital “food”? I have to arrive before the residents and leave after them? And patients/nurses sometimes swat me aside? Really, what is that smell? Have the medical student go figure it out. Oh wait, I am the medical student.

Just remember, you are paying to be used/abused and thrown in the trash. And you have to love it. Why? No reason, you just do.

After the first week, your first patient dies, This is your first clue that it is time to settle in and become the best medical student you can be. I would start by approaching your residents and attending and ask them if the rotation has a syllabus. Most organized programs will have a syllabus and if they don't, you can sit with your superiors and come up with an outline of expectations: what is expected from you and what you are expected to master in the weeks that you are working with them. I would then organize the weeks ahead and try to learn each topic over that period of time. I thought the "Case Files" books were an excellent additive to whatever papers/articles you have to read for each rotation. Case Files have a book for almost each core rotation and they are divided into questions and cases. For me, they were pretty “high yield” and helped with the daily "pimping" and even prepared me well for the USMLE Step 2. But remember, all of the textbooks in the world will not replace the interactions you have with your patients. So please sit and talk to them, get to know them, where they came from, where they are going and, most importantly, how they feel.

So yes, it is true. As a medical student you must show up earliest and leave the latest. It is what it is. Don't fight it. You will lose. Basically from now on it is expected that you sacrifice sleep for medicine. So show up early, get the labs, get the vitals (hopefully your hospital has an EMR otherwise chasing nurses down for charts early in the AM is painful), wake up the patients and ask them how they are (usually angry that you showed up in your little white coat and bothered them) and by the time the resident is there you have all of the info for them. They will adore you and you will almost have a sense of accomplishment. Now the itchy, confusing question about whether or not it is ok to know more about your co-medical students patients than he/she does. Well, yes it is, but please spare us the annoying "know it all" behavior during rounds. If your co-medical student was too busy online dating the night before and doesn't know anything about his patients, you can gently help him out during rounds, but there are more ways to impress the attending without making enemies.

And what about those rotations you cannot stand? For me, it was surgery. Not to say that I don't love the science behind it, but I think my body rejected the idea of waking up early, standing in the cold OR, fighting the residents for an ability to suture, having old, fat surgeon attending yell at me, and never knowing when my next toilet break was. Sometimes you have to fake it until you make it. Oh yes, I definitely did volunteer for each case, yes I did suture all day long and yes I did even consider surgery as a residency (the lack of sleep clouds your sense). But then again, you must go into each rotation knowing that there are many factors that will influence your decision on which specialty to enjoy: the hospital, the residents, the patient population. But if you do understand that u can try to change your perception of a bad rotation and see through the glories of an excellent one.

So now you know what you want to do when you grow up. You have gone through some cores and picked internal medicine (good choice!) and want to ensure you get residency in this complex field. How do you do it? Who do you talk to? Who do you impress? Well, like I mentioned earlier, sit and talk to your attending the first week of your rotation (some will act too cool for school and run away from commitment, but the majority love teaching and will make time for you). Once you know what you want, arrange another meeting and tell them you love internal medicine and hopefully want to focus on women's health, preventive and integrative medicine. What is the best route? Talk to the residents. Not one, not two, not even three, talk to every resident that you cross paths with. What did they do to be accepted into their respective programs? What should you do? Have there been any changes in the requirements in the field? Can they refer you to anyone? And then find your niche within that specialty that you adore and start a research project. Sometimes it will be with an attending/resident in your hospital and sometimes you have to go online and find an attending that is willing to work with you. I have done both and things worked out well for me. Juggling clinical duties and research duties can be daunting, but overall worth it in the end. For me, the addition of research to my clinical work is the most fulfilling part of being a physician and it will allow you to stay current and ahead of the game. So go forward, open those doors in front of you and create your own path in medicine.

Chapter 7

A COLLISION OF EGOS

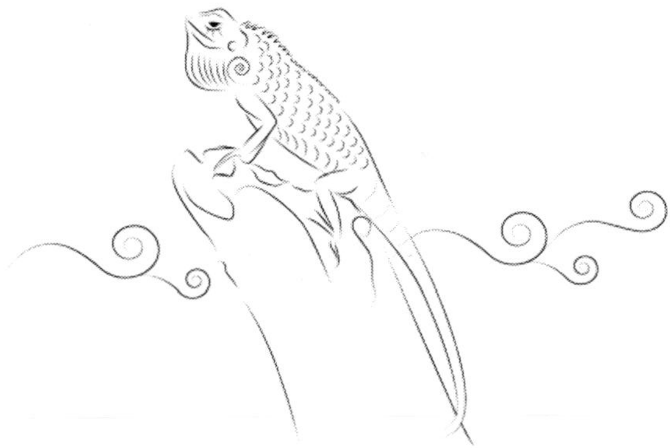

Your time is limited, so don't waste it living someone else's life.
–Steve Jobs

Dr. T

Electives are fun because you basically get to do whatever you are interested in. Creating your own schedule definitely has its ups and downs. For starters, you have to actually decide what it is that you want to do and then you have the challenge of figuring out where you want that experience to take place. It definitely takes a lot of planning and thought. To top it all off you must be strategic in planning because ultimately you need to keep in mind what you want to be when you grow up and what residency program you want to end up in. For example, if you want to do Family Medicine, but have six electives in Cardiac Surgery on your resume then the Family Medicine admissions team may have some concern that you have alternative interests. They may be wondering if Family medicine is just a back up in case you do not match in Cardiac Surgery, for instance.

So that being said, it is important to gear your electives towards your ultimate residency goals. If you want to do Family medicine, for example, then doing your electives not only in family medicine, but also in a variety of other areas is important because everything is relevant to Family Medicine. But, if it's a Surgery residency that you are hoping for, then doing electives relevant to surgery would be important, for example General Surgery, Trauma Surgery, Vascular Surgery, I.C.U. Rotations, Outpatient Surgical Ambulatory Clinics. It's not only which electives that you decide are important, but also where you do them. If you are hoping to do a residency in Canada, it's a no brainer that it would be in your best interest to do your electives in Canada. Similarly, if you want to do your residency at a particular university or hospital, then it might be important to try and arrange elective time at that university or hospital. You want to have the opportunity to work there as a student, not only to familiarize yourself with the hospital, staff and how things run, but also because it's important to meet people and decide if those are the people you want to be your future colleagues.

Electives are also an important times to get reference letters, which are vital to a successful match to a residency program. You want people who got the opportunity to work with you and really get to know you to be writing your reference letters. You want genuine reference letters and not some generic letter that is written by someone you really only worked with once or twice. And you want that letter written by a physician who works in the field you are interested in getting into! In Canada, it's such a small world and when I was at my interviews for Internal Medicine at one university in Ontario, the program director commented that he actually knew the Rheumatologist that wrote my reference letter from British Columbia. Reference letters carry even greater weight when people know and trust the people who are writing them on your behalf.

I did most of my electives across Canada, literally traveling from one side of the country to the other. Because I was initially torn between both Family Medicine and Internal Medicine, I did a variety of electives that were relevant to both specialties including Cardiology, Hematology, Emergency Medicine, Internal Medicine Outpatient Ambulatory Clinic, Pain Management, Family Medicine, Ophthalmology, and Obstetrics and Gynaecology. Most of my electives were either two- or four-week electives. I preferred the four-week electives because I felt like just enough time to really enjoy and appreciate that elective. It always took a good week or so to adjust to a new elective, to figure out your preceptor, what was expected of you, how the new hospital/clinic worked, etc. So, if you only had two weeks and it took you a week to adjust, you really only had a week left before moving on to the next. The longer the elective, the more your preceptor also got to know you and what you were capable of allowing you to get more hands on experience. Longer electives also allow you to follow patients admitted to hospital giving you the opportunity for continuity of care and ultimately better learning.

When you do your electives, you might be the only student working one on one with a preceptor or you may be a part of a team, including a preceptor, residents and other students. Sometimes you will work with students from other Canadian and USA medical schools and sometimes you will work with other international medical graduates. In general, everyone is extremely welcoming and nice. They are happy to have you working with them and as a part of their team. Most people are curious and will ask you questions about where you went to school and your experiences thus far and why you decided to go to a Caribbean Medical school. Occasionally, I had a few snobbish Canadian or USA medical students who think you are getting your medical degree from a cracker-jack box, but they quickly change their perception of you once they realize how well trained you are. In general, and I am not just speaking for myself here, most of the Canadians that I know who went to Ross University get similar, consistent feedback that we are generally harder working and our knowledge is beyond what is expected for our level. It's almost like we have had to fight to get to where we are today and because of that we are always trying extremely hard to prove ourselves to our colleagues that just because we went to a Caribbean Medical school it doesn't mean we are at any disadvantage when it comes to our clinical knowledge and skills.

Electives are fun and give you the opportunity to be exposed to different fields of medicine, which will help you solidify your ultimate decision of what field you want to go into. You meet so many incredible people, and have the opportunity to be exposed to different hospitals/clinics in different cities, provinces and even countries if you want! You not only learn different fields of medicine, but you are exposed to many different styles of practice and different patient populations. Whatever you do, don't waste this precious elective time picking "easy" electives because in the end this is *your* learning opportunity and you will only get out of it what you put into it.

Dr. V

Get a large calendar that covers the whole year(s) and begin filling in important dates. In my case, this calendar covered the wall of my little office and it contained all-important dates. I bought the large erasable calendar because changes occur and often.

It showed my Step exam dates, all core rotation dates, potential elective dates and times to apply. It also showed which school/towns (etc.) I would apply for. So my wall looked like this:

Step 1- date
Cores - 6 dates
Step 2 CS - date/place
Step 2 CK - date/place
Electives: USA/Canada - dates/places
MCCEE -date/place
Apartments - dates/times/places/contacts/contracts

CARMS - application date

It can be overwhelming but if you are well organized, 90% of the battle is done. If you are disorganized, you will be toast. Getting electives in Canada is crucial if you are serious about matching back home. It can be done without Canadian electives, but this is a rare event. I worked hard at getting Canadian electives. I applied on time, completed all paperwork, made many phone calls, and tapped into all possible contacts I could think of in an effort to obtain electives in Canada. All Canadian medical schools have their elective criteria listed on their respective websites. Go to the websites and get familiar with the various processes.

In the end I did electives in Newfoundland, Ontario, Saskatchewan and British Colombia. In the USA, I did electives in Michigan. When I say the paperwork is considerable, what I refer to can be summarized in a cover letter that I used for all of my electives applications in Canada. Here is the actual cover letter reproduced below (this one for Western University - then called UWO); these cover letters were attached to all electives applications:

VANESSA S. DOYLE (MS-4)
P.O. BOX 5000 NEW FEROLLE
NEWFOUNDLAND A0B 4L4
709-846-7560(H) 709-749-2366(C)
VANESSADOYLE@GMAIL.COM

PLEASE FIND ENCLOSED APPLICATION/ DOCUMENTATION FOR ELECTIVES AT UWO

1. APP/APPROVE BY RUSM*
2. IMMUNIZATION RECORDS (UTD)
3. MONEY ORDER/BANK DRAFT
4. RESUME/PASSPORT PHOTO
5. PERSONAL MEDICAL INSURANCE
6. PROOF OF MALPRACTICE INS*
7. CC NON-AFFILIATED FORM

THANK YOU FOR YOUR ATTENTION TO THIS MATTER

VANESSA /12/10/2010

If you send incomplete documentation to the medical schools, it will be filed under Z. If you send a complete professional package to the schools it will be filed under A and taken very seriously. Many people have their applications discarded due to an incomplete application as this adds to the workloads of undergraduate secretaries who try to organize your file for you. Also note under immunization a UTD, this simply means they all have to be Up To Date. Finally, make sure that your email and cell phone number is current and up to date.

When you begin electives, some people will try to make you feel inferior because you are foreign-trained, but as time progresses you begin to realize that your various experiences have taught you so much more than those who are North American trained. We tend to work harder, do not feel entitled, do more grunt work, listen more, learn when we can, stay later, arrive earlier, and have a wider view of the world around us. I mean this sincerely and not just as a pat on the back for IMGs. The hardest part about doing electives in Canada was occasionally dealing with the superiority complex that sometimes reared its head. I have seen my share of divas and prima donnas. Having said that most Canadian-trained medical students are terrific to work with and are very dedicated and exceptional students. But beware, you will meet the divas -- I assure you. This is part of the painful process to building your bridge back to Canada. You have to suck it up, smile politely and move on. What you are really thinking (##%%%%!!!!!!) must always be contained and controlled.

Pick your electives wisely. Make sure you choose areas that interest you. This is where you will get your LORs from Doctors who have worked with you. In my case, I did three electives in Neurology, two in Internal Medicine, and two in Family. The reason being, Neurology was my number one choice Internal was number two, and Family was number three. By the way, always have a back up plan, a plan B when it comes to the match. That planning has to start during your choices for electives.
Put your ultimate goals on that calendar I spoke about earlier. For me, I put in big block letters:

CARMS - NEUROLOGY - INTERNAL MEDICINE - FAMILY MEDICINE.

And never take your eye off the ball, not even for a second. The competition is fierce and so you must use every lever to gain traction and get ahead. Learn to ditch any shyness, be bold and don't be afraid to call, write, phone, or email anyone at anytime for help; everyone competing with you is doing just that.

One final reminder: LORs are obtained during electives and are the MOST IMPORTANT part of your CARMS application. Work hard during electives, get to know your attending, stay late, arrive early and, above all else, ask for that all-important LOR.

Dr. H

Core rotations done, Canadian and American exams done, now it is time for electives, that is, the rotations that I had worked so hard to set-up. As I was determined to come back to Canada for my residency, I planned mostly Canadian electives except for one four week block, which I completed in Michigan.

You may wonder how did I went about setting up these electives? My roommate and I had a two-year calendar outlining our rotations and when we were going to write our exams. We were both determined to come back to Canada for residency. We looked online at all the Canadian universities that allowed international medical graduates to do electives. Then we tentatively put the electives that we wanted on our schedule hoping that we would be able to get approval from the universities for the electives.

The other caveat to applying to all these universities was that each of the schools had their own rules and regulations. For example, there were schools that wanted you to apply nine months in advance of the planned elective. They also had blackout periods where they didn't allow foreign students to rotate through. Having outlined all these rules in our calendars, we applied for each of the electives that we wanted. We also had to submit a form to Ross to approve our electives. These forms, which were very simple and basic, required 30 business days for approval. Ridiculous, right? The age of digital technology and it takes 30 days... It also wasn't as simple as just approving the form. I recall being on the phone so many times to make sure those letters got approved. There was one instance that I will never forget. To apply for my University of Western elective, we had to fill out the form, attach a certified cheque for the cost of the elective and submit it to Ross for approval before it was sent to the University of Western Ontario. I collected all of the forms, including the cheque, and couriered the content to Ross. Several weeks past, but nothing. I was worried and called to follow-up on the progress. Apparently the package had been lost within the Ross building. I couldn't believe what I was hearing. Lost within the building? How was this possible? All that was going through my mind was that I was going to lose my elective spot and how would I get another Canadian certified cheque to send when I was in the states in the middle of my rotation. I was frustrated and angry. Fortunately, I was able to have my husband cancel the old certified cheque and send me another certified cheque. After I put the package together and submit everything to University of Western, I received a call from Ross indicating that they had found the package. Guess where it was all this time? Under the pile of papers on their desk! I was fuming but had to get over it and plan ahead.

With all these ups and downs I still managed to schedule electives at the following universities: University of Toronto, McGill University, University of Western Ontario and University of Winnipeg. I was set to start my journey around Canada. I also had backups electives in the States just in case the Canadian electives didn't come through. Each time I obtained approval from a Canadian school, I would cancel a U.S. elective.

Before I knew it, it was time to the start my first Canadian elective. I was so nervous. I kept thinking, "How will they receive me? Will they think of me less because I was studying abroad?" It wasn't until I was in the rotation that I realized the staff didn't quite care were you were from as long as you worked hard and had good medical knowledge. I remember being praised during my rotations and some thought I was a student from a local medical school. In Canada, as you progress through electives you are given more responsibility to the point that you are functioning as a first-year resident. This was a great experience as it made me really ready for what it was to come in the years ahead and familiar with the Canadian health-care system.

Advice on choosing your electives:

If you are planning on coming back to Canada try and do as much elective as possible within the Canadian health care system. This is important; it will help you when you apply for CARMS. Also, if possible try and do electives in hospitals you would like to work in eventually. Work hard during your electives and don't let people think you are inferior because you studied abroad. Choose your electives wisely, it will reflect what you would like to do in the future and you don't want to just fill it with anything.

Dr. R

Congratulations! You have made it to your fourth year of medical school. Only four to 10 years left and maybe $300,000 in loans to pay off, but really you should be so proud! You have gone where no sane person has gone before and now it is time to choose (at least choose within the choices presented) exactly whom you are going to learn from and where the learning will take place. Elective rotations serve exactly that purpose and many more: they are rotations you choose in your fourth year of medical school, so make sure you choose them carefully. Here is my advice:

- Some electives are just "chill", essentially "vacation rotations" where you show up, smile (in my case try to smile), answer three to four questions from the attending and then go. Not really that easy but you get the point.
- Other electives are important for your career, i.e. rotations that are not cores but considered important, like anesthesia, plastic surgery, ICU, neurology or sub-specialty electives in the program that you may be considering (e.g. a cardiology elective if you are considering internal medicine).
- Electives are also an excellent tool to help you explore other areas of medicine (e.g. if you are applying for anesthesiology,

it may benefit your mind and soul to take some electives in paediatric and/or internal medicine).

- Some choose elective time for research opportunities, which not only makes you a much better physician, but also helps you network and build your resume.
- And last, but definitely not least, electives are the best way for you to "interview" the potential hospital in which you wish to obtain residency.

Electives are usually two to four weeks long and it is within this short time span that you get to see the hospital in a light that you would never be able to see if you only interviewed there. Each hospital tries its hardest to present themselves in the best way they can on interview day, but we all know each program has its pitfalls (dirty call rooms, poor sub-specialty support, lack of research, absent attending, horrible cafeteria food, lack of support from the program director). Some of these items may not seem important, but believe me if you are eating sludge for breakfast, lunch and dinner, it does make a difference – both for your health and for those who have to endure your burrito breath. At the same time, this is a chance for the hospital to scope you out and determine whether they like you or not. So yes, electives are generally "chill" unless you really want to impress and really want to be a part of the program. I hassled the programs I was interested in, but took a chill pill during my anesthesia and plastics rotations.

I started developing an idea of where I wanted to do my electives during the early part of my third year of medical school. I chose some based on location and others based on program. I started applying midway (yes, you have to apply for some electives) during my third year and there were places I was not accepted to -- some due to timing, some because they didn't like my application (how dare they!), and others because they don't take foreign grads – it is true.

Overall, I found a healthy balance of electives and a lot of mine were away electives in internal medicine. I did electives in Santa Barbara, New York City, Miami and the city of dreams: LA. I even got accepted to do electives at the University of Toronto, but unfortunately had to turn it down because I knew I wanted to do residency in the States (specifically, California) and I was also busy studying for the multitude of board exams. I remember applying for electives and thinking to myself that I wished I could do all the electives in the world!

Chapter 8

CHASING RESIDENCY

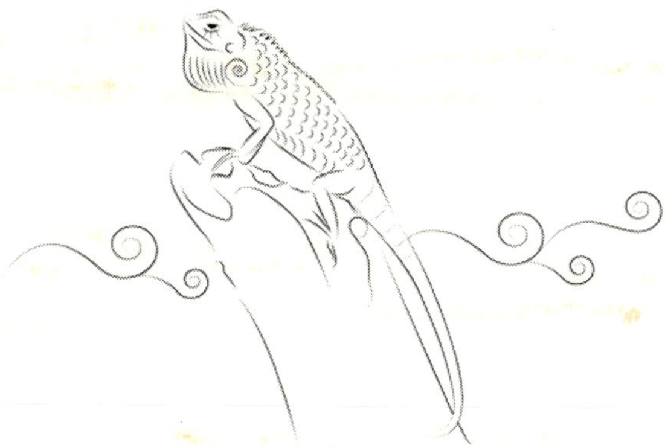

The question isn't who is going to let me; it's who is going to stop me.

–Ayn Rand

Dr. T

I only applied to CaRMS (Canadian Residency Matching Service). I thought long and hard about the decision to only apply to residency in Canada, but I had to be realistic and honest with myself about my future goals. I wanted to be back home in Canada, closer to my family. I planned to practice in Canada and thus it was important to me to also have my residency training in Canada. I was definitely taking a huge risk by not applying to match in the USA. I am an International Medical Graduate and my potential residency spots are limited both in Canada and the USA. I had to think about the possibility that if I did not match in Canada, I would not be starting ANY residency programs next year!

Canadians that apply to both Canada and the USA have the advantage of finding out if they matched in Canada first, so that they can be removed from the US match if they obtain a spot in Canada.

Likewise, if they do not match in Canada, they will still be in the running to match in the USA as a back up.

CaRMS is a typical application process much like the one that you filled out to get into medical school. You will create your own CARMS file online and it will include all of your basic personal information, as well as all of the details of your educational and personal endeavors. The most important part about the whole process is listing the programs that you are interested in applying to and reading through each program-specific application requirements. Every university and each program has its own application requirements. They will each specify exactly what kind and how many reference letters they are looking for. They will all have different guidelines and expectations for writing a personal letter. Yes, that means you will end up writing a different personal letter for each program! Very time consuming, but very important! Don't make the mistake of writing a generic letter that you send to all programs because, trust me, they will notice when reading them (Yes – the programs actually read your letters!). Remember to be strategic with which program you send each reference letter to. You may have acquired many different reference letters and some may be the perfect letter for one program, but another may more appropriate for the next program. For example, if you are applying to Surgery and you have acquired a reference letter from a Nephrologist and another from a Surgeon you did an elective with, you will probably want opt for the letter from the surgeon – at least when applying to a surgery residency. You must submit all of your documents to CaRMS, which will then appear in your online file, and then you can go through each program requirement and attach the right files to each specific program.

You need to be organized and remember to be aware of the different deadlines. All of the information you need is on the CaRMS website. If you have questions or need help with anything, I recommend calling the CaRMS support staff. They are fabulous and it's best to call them with your questions rather than go by hearsay from other students. Oh and of course there is a fee. Basically the more programs you apply for, the more it costs!

Being an international medical graduate, I applied to basically every single Family Medicine and Internal Medicine program that I was eligible to apply to across the country. I was so determined to get back to Canada that I didn't really care where I went. I was ready to move anywhere in Canada if it meant I got the opportunity to do residency in Canada! Obviously I had a preference. There were certain programs that appealed to me more than others, but when I was at the initial stage of application, I didn't want to limit my options. I guess that's another point I should make: when you are deciding what programs you want to apply to check out their programs website and actually take some time to read and learn about the program. Jot down your pros and cons for each program and take note of the curriculum, elective opportunities, scheduled academic learning time, research opportunities and anything else that you might value about a program.

I applied to both Family Medicine and Internal Medicine. When the applications came out in the fall, I was still undecided between the two specialties. I loved them both and because I was still undecided I did not want to limit my options. Interviews were not until January and February, so I wanted to give myself more time to decide. Remember you will be doing this for the rest of your life! The only downside of applying to multiple specialties is that it costs more and of course it creates more work because more programs mean more personal letters to write, etc. Programs do not know how many specialties or programs you applied to and so you don't need to worry that it will look bad if you apply to multiple places.

The whole process is admittedly nerve-racking, overwhelming and exhausting! Remember, you are still doing rotations during this time. So not only are you studying or preparing presentations for the clinical rotation you are currently doing, you have to come home and write personal letters, edit them, edit them again and edit them one final time. It's a lot of work! My word of advice: spend the quality time you need to do your applications and ask a friend or family to help you edit your personal letters, curriculum vitae, etc. Be aware of deadlines and get started early so that you are not rushing around trying to crunch and make a deadline. Do your research on the programs and write your personal letters to reflect that. Like I said, generic personal letters are obvious to the reader.

The best part about the whole process is hitting submit! What a relief it is when you finally hit submit. Soon you will be anxiously waiting by your Smartphone for the emails start coming through -- hopefully inviting you to an interview!

Dr. V

Chasing residency requires determination dedication perseverance and above all strategy.
I could have applied to both the USA and Canada, but I chose only Canada because that's where I wanted to be. It was a risk, but one I was prepared to take.

My own personal strategy was to "go long and go wide". What I mean by that is my focus was to cover as many provinces as I could and to target at least three disciplines. So in terms of provinces, I focused on Newfoundland, Nova Scotia, Ontario, Manitoba and Saskatchewan. For programs, my focus was Neurology, Internal and Family.

Interviews always happen in mid-January and early February so plan to be traveling during this time. Remember, it's winter, so be ready. Book Air Canada flight passes that can be used anytime and flight changes (which will happen) are free. When my application was completed and filed, I waited for emails inviting me for interviews. Here is what my interview schedule looked like in 2012 match:

Interviews
1. FRIDAY, JAN. 20 @ 8:00 a.m.: FM- ONTARIO: Mine was scheduled at U of T, but you can do yours at any of the sites.

2. MONDAY, JAN. 23 @ 8:00 a.m.: NEURO- MANITOBA

3. FRIDAY, JAN. 27 @ 3:00 p.m.: IM- OTTAWA

4. SATURDAY, JAN. 28 @ 8:00 a.m.: FM- DAL (I missed

because of a storm...yes this is reality when you live in Canada and CARMS interviews are this time of year...if you miss an interview, even if it's out of your control, tough luck!)

5. MONDAY, JAN. 30 @ 12:10 p.m.: NEURO- UWO

6. WEDNESDAY, Feb. 1 @ 2:00 p.m.: NEURO- OTTAWA

7. FRIDAY, FEB. 3 @ 4:30 p.m.: IM- UWO

8. TUESDAY, FEB. 7: TELEPHONE INTERVIEW: FM-MANITOBA (I cancelled a few days prior since I had little interest in residency there and my interviews in neurology and IM, which I preferred, were going really well)

9. USASK - Family Medicine (I cancelled a few days prior since I had little interest in residency there, and I was exhausted from the CARMS tour by that time)

10. MUN - Family medicine (I attended, since I was there doing an elective, but ranked last since they didn't offer me an interview initially until I inquired as to why I was not offered an interview, being from NL and having completed 12 weeks of electives there...I mean really MUN....someone from Toronto is really likely to stay in NL after residency?!?!)

11. Dal - Internal Medicine (I cancelled after I read the fine print, that says you cannot sub-specialize, you can only go general IM, which did not appeal to me, plus it's discriminating against IMGs!)

Here are some up-to-date and very insightful thoughts from a fellow Ross grad who entered the 2014 match.

His CaRMS journey: (Dr. K. Morgan - PGY 1 - Ottawa)

Step 2 CS Dec 5th - Finished core rotations

Feb 22, 2013 - took Step 2 CK
Mar 16, 2013 - MCCEE Mar 21, 2013 (reviewed community health section of Toronto Notes and did as many questions as possible on Canada Q bank)

Sept 2013 - NAC -OSCE
Oct 2013 - MMI
Nov 2013 - MCCQE1

- 2 FM electives in Canada (Ottawa and Western) – These were difficult to get. I made sure my application was there the first day applications were being accepted and followed with multiple phone calls. I was always pleasant with the administrators and befriended them. They are the gateway to your electives.

- While doing my elective in Ottawa, they informed me that their internal cutoff for interviews/ranking for Ottawa FM was 380 on the EE. All schools are not the same.

- Had 4 LORs from Canadian physicians.

- Family Medicine Interviews: Applied to Ontario/Manitoba/Saskatchewan/Alberta
  Interviews granted:
  Ontario Joint FM (6 programs)
  Manitoba Joint FM (4 programs)
  Saskatoon
  Regina
  U of Calgary (AIMG program)
  U of Alberta (AIMG program)

- Internal Medicine: Applied to Ottawa/Western/Toronto/Calgary
  Two of four interviews granted:
  U of Toronto
  U of Calgary

- Ranked 19 programs in Canada
  Ranked 8 programs in USA

EXAMS

MCCEE

- 180 questions, 150 scored
- Relatively "easy" compared to Step 2 CK, but cannot be taken lightly. It is VERY easy to pass, but if you want any chance of matching in Canada, you need to get a score over 370 (in my opinion).
- Some very ambiguous questions, short stems. Much less clear the Step 2 CK questions.
- lost a couple points due to Canadian-specific content (drug names).
- Resources: whatever you used to prepare for Step2 CK plus doing Canada question bank is helpful (although inferior to UWorld or Kaplan, it can help get a few questions that are Canadian specific.) Community health/public health/ethics section of Toronto Notes.

Nac OSCE

- Similar to Step 2 CK, but more challenging.
- Before the clinical stations there is a multiple-choice exam of 30 questions x 30 minutes long. It is a random assortment of questions from every discipline. Doses of medications are not required knowledge (they used to be).
- 12 stations -- 11 are scored/1 pilot station.
- 11 minutes long, 2 min between stations, same format as Step 2 CS.
- 8 minutes given for the objectives outlined when you walk in room (history/physical/ history and counseling, etc).
- 3 minutes (after buzzer)- examiner questions. Questions vary widely from differential diagnosis, management plans, and interpretation of radiographs. This can be tricky because a point might have a large DDx, but there is little time for reorganizing information in your head. Many rooms require counseling patients, this is how they measure your communication skills, which is important for this exam.
- Make sure to read instructions carefully, because each station asks you to complete different tasks and you don't want to do

a physical when you don't have to (and you will run out of time).

- You must talk out loud about what you are doing when doing physical exam. This is to let them know what you are looking for. Points allocated accordingly.
- No note required when you leave room (major difference from CS).
- Examiner is in the room; they monitor your clinical skill techniques.
- There is one room that may have an "emergency" situation. Make sure to ask for vitals and do a quick, focused history and a comprehensive physical exam. The section in resource below covers this well.

Examples of rooms I experienced:
1. Cranial nerve exam
2. Left arm radiculopathy
3. Chest pain
4. Lower back pain/drug seeker
5. Volume status assessment
6. Newborn jaundice
7. Teen Abdominal pain
8. Pneumothorax

Resources: NAC OSCE – A comprehensive review by Canada prep is a worthwhile resource to buy. It covers the 30-question therapeutics section well. Also a good review of some physical exams that are not covered in First Aid Step 2CS. Only shortcoming is it is not a question/answer based case review.

Spend time learning the management parts of the clinical cases. Although I did well on this exam, I felt this was where I was weaker and should have spent more time preparing. The new version of this text may be out soon. I used version 1.

Thank you Dr K.

Be patient when filing your application for the CaRMS match and follow the milestones carefully. Make sure that you don't leave the ROL to the last minute.

And never doubt your choices!

Dr. H

I'm a fourth year medical student. It's the last year that I'm going to pay tuition. Next year I'm going to earn money after a very long time of not getting paid.

This marks the scary time of the year where all the medical students begin to fear where they will find themselves next year. Will we match to the programs that we want; will we be in the location that we want. I was terrified. As an international medical graduate, I knew it was going to be hard to land a residency position in Canada, as there were only a few spots available.

After going through most of my rotations I knew that I wanted to apply to both Internal Medicine and Family Medicine for residency. I had decided to apply to both the United States and Canada because I wanted to make sure I had a residency spot. I was too afraid to only apply to Canada for residency just in case I didn't match.

Now that I had made the decision to apply to both systems, it was time to fill out the applications. To be honest, the NRMP (National Resident Matching Program) process was so complicated and poorly organized that I don't remember much of it. I think that my brain has blocked most of it out, as the experience was so unpleasant. As I was filling out the application, I thought to myself that I only want to go to one hospital for my residency if I don't get into Canada. So based on this, I only filled out the application for the one hospital that I was interested in. I also did an elective at this hospital; this being the only elective that I did outside of Canada during my fourth year. While I was doing my elective, I was interviewed for a residency spot and was offered a position for the following year. I was thrilled with the offer. But I still really wanted to give Canada a chance. I had to decline the pre-match and ask them to rank me, as Canada was my first choice based on proximity to family. I was lucky that they understood where I was coming from and the hospital accepted the option of ranking me in order to allow me to go through the Canadian matching system.

As for the CaRMS experience, this was much more pleasant. As international medical graduates, we had to write one extra exam before being eligible to apply for Canadian residency. The exam is called MCCEE. You have to write this exam as a Canadian whether you decide to apply to a Canadian residency or not, but the score you get matters if you want to apply to CaRMS. I wrote this exam when I wrote my USMLE Step 2 CK as the exam material were very similar.

To participate in CaRMS, you need to register and get a token to start your application. When the time came I obtained my token and started my application. This application is very similar to a medical school application. You fill in the basic information, where you studied, what rotations you have completed, research, and work experience. It also allows you to upload documents that are needed for each university that you apply to. CaRMS is not like the NRMPs rolling admission. There is a deadline and after that all the applications get reviewed at once and then interviews are offered. I started to work on my application at the beginning of the summer, taking my time to make sure each section was filled out as best as possible. I learned from other Canadian students how to input my elective and describe the skills I acquired during my rotations. I spent months working on my personal statement, making sure it was how I wanted to portray myself to the admission committee. I had everyone read my personal statement to make sure it was perfect and without error. When doing electives try and see if there are residents who are willing to read and comment on your personal statement. They have been through it and at times have done these interviews and are able to give great advice.

The hardest part of the application process was collecting of reference letters. You have to strategically select supervisors who will write a stellar letter. You want them to highlight what makes you a better resident over the other candidates. If they write a standard letter it works against you during the application review process. This is important, since you are ranked on your reference letters. One way you to make sure you pick the right supervisors are to select the ones who give you the best feedback or the ones who offer to write you a letter. If you are not sure, ask them and if they hesitate, you won't want them to write your reference letter.

In order to ensure the letters get to CaRMS on time, provide your references with prepaid mailing packages. I provided each reference with a prepaid express mailing package. I figured they were already taking time out of their busy schedules to write a letter that the least I could do was provide them with prepaid postage. I also wanted to make sure the letters got to CaRMS as quickly as possible.

Planning is key to completing your applications accurately and on time. You need to make sure you read everything and plan which documents need to be sent and by when, so that you won't miss the deadlines. I planned out when everything had to be in to CaRMS and made sure I was on schedule. This includes everything from writing the exam at the most appropriate time, which supervisors to ask to do my reference letters and when.

Nevertheless, this is a stressful time in your medical school career. There is so much uncertainty that it can drive you crazy. I had worked so hard throughout my rotations and even harder on my exams to make sure I had the best foot forward. I already knew it was going to be hard as an international medical graduate to secure a spot; I didn't want to have any further holdbacks. The application deadline came and I submitted my application to CaRMS. Then I prayed that I would land interviews in Canada.

Now that the applications were in, all I had to do was wait. I knew that by the middle of December, they would announce if we had landed an interview or not. I was counting the days and as mid-December drew closer, the more nervous I became. What if I didn't get any interviews? What would I do then? I didn't want to be away from my husband for another three years. I was tired of long-distance relationships.

It was finally mid-December and I recall the sweet email that read, "Congratulations, you have been invited for an interview for family medicine". I was driving with my husband and was so happy when I saw the email. Yes, I made it through the first step. I quickly selected the locations where I would like to interview, hoping that I would land Toronto as number one. As the month moved along, I started to get invitations to other locations that I had applied to. At the end I had interviews for family medicine at all the schools in Ontario, University of Halifax and University of Winnipeg, and internal medicine interviews at University of Western Ontario, McMaster University and University of Ottawa. I had two weeks booked off for the interviews and bought my tickets. I was moving from one city to the next with very little time in between. I was ready to travel; now it was time to prepare myself for the interviews.

I got in touch with an organization in Toronto called Health Force Ontario. The organization helps international medical graduates prepare for interviews and land a job. I attended their seminars on how to prepare for interviews. They went over the types of questions that could be asked and how to answer the questions to make sure you highlight why you are the best candidates for the position. After the seminar, I booked mock-interviews with the advisors. I dressed like it was an actual interview and went in hoping for the best. They asked questions and I answered. During the process I kept thinking, "I'm not doing badly". It wasn't till the end when we were debriefing that they pointed out all the things I needed to improve on and how to best answer questions.

I took their advice and corrected the mistakes and did two more mock-interviews with them. Once that was done, I took all the sample questions and wrote out all the answers along with examples that I would use during the interview. Then I just kept rehearsing the questions until I felt ready. I was determined to land a residency in Canada and was going to make sure I was very prepared for my interviews.

The time came and it was the day before my first interview: Family Medicine in Toronto. I was so nervous. I had my suit picked out and dress shirt ironed. I went over all the questions and my answers again. I tried to get a good night sleep but let's be honest, who can get a good night sleep before an interview that will potentially determine your future. I managed to sleep for a few hours and woke up really early getting ready. I needed to travel to the location without getting stuck in Toronto traffic. I left so early that I was super early for my interview. When I got to the building it wasn't me who was nervous after all, there were many more candidates who had arrived as early as I did. You could see the nervousness in each of them. When the time came we were escorted up to the level and the room where we waited before being called for the interview. I was so nervous, but tried to conquer my nerves by talking to other candidates. Who knew, maybe we would be colleagues one day.

I heard my name called and was then told which door to go through for the interview. The next half hour was a blur and it went by so fast. All I remember is that I made sure to highlight the breadth of my experience and qualifications and why I would be a great resident and should be ranked high. I recall exiting the interview and not knowing how it went, but still felt (a bit) relieved that it was over. I had to keep focusing on the other interviews ahead.

The days went by and I finished one interview after another. I travelled with the same group of people from one interview to the next. We were all from different schools, but shared the same goal of landing a residency spot in Canada.

The most interesting interview was for Family Medicine in Halifax. The interview consisted of 12 stations of mini-interview questions where you debated with another resident, gave directions or answered a question. It was my first time through an interview of this sort. I was nervous but found it very interesting and intriguing.

As I went through my interviews, I felt glad that I had spent time arranging Canadian electives and had Canadian references. This was especially beneficial, as some of the interviewers knew the supervisors that I had worked with and that I was familiar with the Canadian health system. My desire to land residency in Canada was clear.

After finishing my interviews it was time to rank them. I had been given the advice of rank where you want to go and not how you felt on your interview because that is not accurate. I had to decide which university and program I wanted to go to. I had applied to both Family Medicine and Internal Medicine residency positions. I found this part difficult because I didn't just have to think about what I wanted, but how my decision would affect my relationship with my husband and our lives. We had been long distance through all my schooling; would we have to be long distance through my residency as well? After much soul-searching and discussion with friends and colleagues, I decided to rank schools based on proximity to home and what I wanted my life to be. I knew I wanted to have family and work–life balance, and the only profession that would allow me to have both was family medicine. My rank list was complete and after going over it many times, I finally submitted it. The waiting game began. Match day was March 7 and I would have to wait to see where I would go.

I counted the days till Match day, as any other anxious medical student does. March 7 arrived and I was glued to my computer from morning to lunch when I received that infamous email saying you can access to see your match results. My hands were shaking as I was navigating through the web browser and entering my password. My heart was beating so hard and I held my breath as the final page loaded. As I scrolled down the page, I read "Congratulations you have been matched to University of Toronto Family Medicine". I couldn't believe it. I read it again and again and then it finally sunk in. I jumped up and down screaming, "I matched, I matched". I was ecstatic. I told my partner and family the great news and let the celebration start.

Dr. R

Your fourth year of medical school should be enjoyed. Although it was one of the most stressful times of my life, I managed to travel around the country, learn a ton from sub-specialists, visit different hospitals and, yes, I managed to fit in 18 residency interviews. I am not going to lie, I was fat, furious and pimply, but I got it done!

I have many nicknames for myself, but the one that suits me the most is "gypsy girl". My name, Raheleh, means "traveler". I have always had the itch to move and continue moving. "Entropy" is what it is called in science; "childish" is what my mom says; "the good life" is what my friends say; but for me, I am a "modern day gypsy". The modern day gypsy enjoys all the luxuries of a stable life (a home, a shower, no criminal record) but at the same time is able to experience the wings of freedom. And so when the time came to apply for residency I knew that I wanted something new. To live in a place that I had not previously lived and so why not a different country? So I didn't bother with CaRMS and stuck to NRMP (National Resident Matching Program). I also remember two distinct conversations I had with a friend (who is an MD) and an attending at a hospital in LA. Both were Canadian and both practiced emergency medicine. My friend was shocked when I told him how frequently I saw gunshot wounds in the ER as he had never seen one before during his career as an attending and/or medical student. I relayed this information to the Canadian attending working in LA and he smirked, "Canadians don't know how to have fun. I moved here for the good stuff." "My goodness," I bet you are exclaiming. How can she want to see gunshot wounds? No, I don't want to see gunshot wounds, I don't want to see people hurt, but the reality is that it exists and if I can learn to deal with it than I will be an amazing physician. The truth is that there are more people in the United States; more people mean more disease, more disease means pathology, more pathology makes for a better clinician.

Applying for NRMP was expensive, time consuming and something I never want to deal with again. The hardest part of medical school is the paperwork you have to deal with over and over again. There is a list of things that must be submitted prior to applying. You must go on the NRMP website and step by step go through the process of application. I could rant on and on about every item, but that would be a fruitless venture. Let me boil it down to the things I feel a lot of student's mess up:

- LORs – oh the dreaded letters of recommendation. Who has the nerve to approach an attending and ask for a letter? It is the worst. But you gotta do what you gotta do to survive. And believe me all attendings have templates for all you medical students (unless you are uber exceptional and they will write one specifically for you). You must ask soon and collect these LORs. Obviously ERAS wants them to be confidential and to this day I still disagree with this, but some attendings will show you your LOR. However, nowadays you youngers are required to do everything electronically, so LORS are uploaded straight from your attending computer to ERAS. Back in my day, we had to cut down trees to make the paper and take the horse and buggy over to the hospital...

- Personal statements: I love reading these. I think I have read and re-read at least 20-30 since I got accepted into residency. They are hard to write. Let's be real, you must sum up your crazy reasoning for giving up a real life and entering medical school in less than two pages. (Ideally one page). Are you kidding me? No I am not. It is essentially your personal statement for medical school, but more refined. Remember you now have MD following your name. Submission date: it boggles my mind why people always ask when to submit their applications? Especially FMGs! The answer is the day ERAS opens submissions. End of story. Stop asking. I said stop asking!
- Can I apply to more than one program (i.e. internal medicine, family medicine)? Yes you can, but be careful if you decide to apply to more than one program within the same hospital, especially when it comes to small hospitals. People talk and if they see you at the General Surgery interview and the week before you were interviewing for Psychiatry, they may not take your interest in the program seriously. Can you blame them? My recommendation is to find something that sparks your interest and apply to that. Applying at random only means you don't know what you want...and I guess that makes you a woman?
- How many programs to apply to? This is a tough one to answer. It depends entirely on what you are applying for, how strong your application is and are you willing to live in the middle of nowhere? Apparently I was. I have a healthy sense of paranoia mixed with a determination to make it happen so I applied to 100 programs. In retrospect, did I need to do this? No. But it eased my conscience and I ended up attending 18 interviews (and saw villages such as Saginaw, Michigan).

Once you apply, sit back and wait… and wait. You may get a rejection right away or you may get an interview. Don't be discouraged! It takes a while to eventually get a collection of interviews that you want. You may even have to turn some down (I did). And where to get all the bling to make these interviews happen? For me it was student loans. Some people may be lucky enough and their parents will support them, but the majority will rely on loans. I learned to live a frugal life sans mani-pedis, fine wines, trips around the world. Ok, whom am I kidding? I managed to fit that in somehow. But it was hard. As Thomas Edison once said "There is no substitute for hard work." Don't let anyone tell you otherwise. Being a first generation Canadian I am proud to say I learned hard work, perseverance and courage from my parents (but don't tell them I said this).

Tips for the interview day:

- What to wear: dress conservatively. I wore a basic black suit and had alternating shirts that matched. Wear comfortable shoes because you will be doing a lot of walking. I alternated between dressy flats and very comfortable wedges.
- How to act: Be normal. We all know you are not, but attempt it during interview season. Smile, be gracious, eat slowly and mindfully, ask questions with your hand raised, don't take over and be aggressive, don't be a know-it-all, don't be rude or annoying, don't chew gum, don't use your cell to check Facebook. Basically, you should behave like a civilized human. For me, this was the hardest part.
- How to travel: Make sure to ask the program if they offer hotels or discounts at the minimum. I took trains, planes, buses, walked, drove during the interview season. I figured out the most economical means to travel the country and had minimal breakfast, free lunch during the interview and generally ate small dinners.
- Questions to ask: There are a multitude of questions you may ask and contrary to popular belief there is such a thing as a stupid question. So don't embarrass yourself, but at the same time be genuine. Ask about residency wellness (i.e. are they happy, do they get along); ask about the food, sub-specialty services, etc.

- How to follow-up: An email to both the program director and the person interviewing should be sufficient. It is important to thank them for their time and be sure to include why you wish to match at their program.

It's time to rank!

- How to rank: It may seem difficult to realize this, but really the match works in your favor and you should rank the programs based on where you want to match, not where you think you are going to match.

Lastly as a Canadian you need a statement of need from the Government of Canada. This is a formal letter from the government of your citizenship, which states the dire need of physicians needed in your home country. Sadly, Canada makes you take a board exam prior to issuing you this letter. Make sure to register for this exam around the same time as you prepare for Step 2. This exam is only offered twice per year and if you end up missing it even if you match you cannot start your residency.

Chapter 9

THE REAR VIEW MIRROR

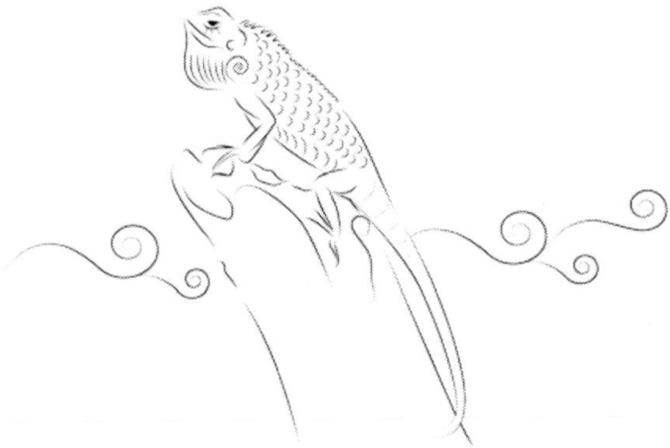

"It's kind of fun to do the impossible."

- Walt Disney

Dr. T

After submitting your application, it is a hard waiting game. I remember being hyper vigilant for any phone beep or sound. Immediately checking any and all alerts on my phone indicating that an email had been received. All invitations received for interviews came by email. It was a very exciting time. For me, I was fortunate to get most invitations for interviews. I did, however, get a few dreaded emails telling me in a polite way that I was not chosen for an interview. Oh well, you win some you lose some!

Next begins the crazy task of booking all your interviews. Each program has a specific day or days on which they hold their interviews. The interviews are often accompanied by some sort of tour and social event with the current residents. It becomes the craziest few weeks of your life as you find yourself booking multiple flights all over the country, sometimes trying to figure out a way to make back-to-back interviews. Remember interview time is just a few weeks in January and February: the middle of winter! And while booking flights is a challenge, the weather is out of your control. It seems like there are always the maddest winter storms smack in the middle of the interview weeks. If you miss an interview due to a cancelled or delayed flight, tough luck! I didn't make it to Manitoba because I couldn't get out of Newfoundland on time, but they did offer me a phone interview in lieu of the in-person interview. (As you can imagine a phone interview is just not the same as one in person.) And you think you are a broke, starving student already? Or you just finished paying off that application fee on your credit card? Well, flying is not free and neither are accommodations. Be prepared for all costs associated with the interviews. I shared hotel rooms with my friend who had a similar schedule as me in order to save money. Plus, it is way more fun to travel and explore new cities with a friend!

Remember, you may have applied to multiple programs and specialties and now a few months later have decided that you are not interested in a certain program anymore. Be honest with yourself and communicate that message to the program. Don't waste your time, your money or the interviewers time by going to an interview if you don't plan on ranking them in your final list.

Interview season as they call it is a fun few weeks. While you are travelling around the country with your head cut off, you are often doing it with the same group of candidates. You meet amazing people and the program socials are always a lot of fun. The socials are usually filled with current residents who are welcoming, fun and easy to talk to. They are your best source of information for all questions you might not want to ask a program director. Are the residents happy? How is the social life? Are they a family friendly program? What are the strengths and weaknesses of the program? What would they change about their program? It is also an opportunity for you to check out who your future colleagues might be. Are they the type of people you could and would want to work with? Could these people be your friends? Social events are usually at some sort of restaurant or bar and there is often yummy food and drinks. I think it's important to try accommodate your travel plans to include the social if possible. I missed a couple socials simply because of back-to-back interviews and while I would have loved to go, it is not the end of the world if you miss them. The socials are not part of your interview and have absolutely no weight on your interview score.

Interviews are pretty similar across the board. Most are either one-on-one with a program director or staff, or a panel of the program director, staff and a current resident. To my surprise, most interviews are very casual in the sense that they really just want to know who you are and why you are right for the program and why the program is right for you. There are the usual standard interview questions, but I felt like most interviews were more of a conversation. The interviewers have often already read your entire application and so they don't need you to reiterate all the wonderful things you have done. They may be interested in learning more about specific things you have in your application.

I went to one interview that was not your usual interview – it consisted of multiple mini-interviews. There were multiple stations that you rotated through. Some stations asked you to perform or complete a specific task and some stations were more interview style question asking. It's kind of fun to do the multiple mini-interviews because if you feel like you mess up at one station, you still have several other stations to make a good impression.

My advice would be to ensure you prepare for your interview with a friend or family member. Don't rehearse and memorize your answers because it doesn't sound natural. More importantly, think about popular interview questions. For instance: What are your strengths? What are your weaknesses? Why this program? Why you? Have an idea about what you want to say so you are not stuck or put on the spot. Make sure you do a little reading about the program prior to the interview so that you can ask appropriate questions and tailor some of your answers to their program. Most importantly, be yourself! Be polite, smile, take a deep breath and have fun. If you made it to an interview you have already made it through the hardest part. The people who are interviewing you just want to get to know you a bit as a person and are deciding in their heads if they can picture you as a colleague. They are deciding whether or not they want to work with you.

I was asked one medical question at one of my interviews; it was a fairly simple question, but may catch you off-guard. Pause, take a deep breath and think about it. I like to repeat the question out loud and talk aloud through my solution. Don't let it throw you off. The hardest interview question I was asked was "If you had three special powers, what would they be and why?" This one definitely stumped me because I definitely had not prepared myself for that one. I am pretty sure my answers were horrible. I didn't want to sound cliché and save the world or end world hunger (even though I do!), so I think I said something like I would want a magic flying carpet or something weird like that. Bottom line: be yourself, prepare and have fun! Of course, dress and act professional. By the way, everyone wears black suits; it looks like you are all at a funeral. Not saying that you should wear something crazy and stand out, just pointing out the obvious.

After all the interviews are over, it's time to make a gigantic list with all the pros and cons of each program. Which program is the ideal fit for you? What is important to your decision? Is it location, curriculum, research Opportunity, opportunity for fellowship, etc.? There is a lot to think about and if you have a partner or family, it's really important you include them in your decision. In the end you, have the daunting task of putting all the programs in a ranked order of your number one choice all the way down to your last choice. You don't have to rank a program if you absolutely do not want to go there. Remember that you may get your fifth or tenth choice and you want to make sure that you are happy with those choices as well.

Looking back it was definitely the adventure of a lifetime! Every sleepless on-call night, daunting exam, 4 a.m. morning rounds during my surgery rotation, rectal exams... it was all worth it. I am where I am today because of this crazy adventure and I couldn't be happier.

I feel like I am a better doctor today because of everything that I have been so lucky to experience. I was very fortunate to have been exposed to such a variety of patients, pathology and healthcare systems and ways of practicing medicine. I have met some of the most wonderful people, magnificent mentors, and made some of my greatest lifelong friends. I have travelled and lived in many places and this alone comes with countless memories and experiences.

There are two things I would change if I had to do it again. For starters, I would have applied to more medical schools across Canada. I only applied to the University of British Columbia, but I often wonder if I had applied to other medical schools in Canada if I would have been accepted. Not that I would trade my experience for any other, but going to medical school in Canada would have been a whole lot cheaper! And let's be honest here, things are just easier when you graduate from a Canadian Medical School. As an International medical graduate, you face a few extra challenges and steps along the way. You need to write additional exams, there's often more paperwork to fill out for things like electives and residency applications, and it's generally more competitive and challenging to get a residency spot. International Medical Graduates also have Return of Service Agreements with the province in which they do their residency. For example, because I did my residency in Ontario, I have to give back five years of service in Ontario before I can practice anywhere else in the country. These Return of Contract agreements also have specific rules about where in the province you can work and how long you can locum for, etc. Canadian medical graduates don't have these kinds of restrictions. But, at the end of the day, I would not change my medical adventure for the world. Besides, if I did get into a Canadian medical school, I am sure I would have excelled and loved it just as much only I would never know what I missed out on!

The other thing I would change if I were to do it again would be to have done rotations in a few more cities in the States, such as Florida or New York. I think it would have been cool to live in these places and explore them during one of my rotations. When else in my life will I have the opportunity to live and work for a short time in these great cities? That being said, because I was on a strict, frugal student budget, I was happy stay in one spot and pay rent in Michigan rather then move to New York City and pay some ridiculously overpriced short-term rental rate. Also staying in one city for a majority of your rotations has many additional advantages simply because you don't have to move every four weeks and you really get to know your community and hospital.

Well, there you have it folks. A snapshot of my crazy medical school adventure. If you are thinking of applying to medical school, then I wish you the very best of luck. Do your research and find the school that you think suits you best. Whether you stay in your home province or state or venture to another university within your country or decide to study abroad, at the end of the day you are going to ultimately reach your end goal of becoming a physician. However you choose to get there is up to you! If you are currently in medical school, then what are you doing reading this book? You don't have time to read for pleasure, so get back to studying or, better yet, use your time wisely and sleep! But I guess if you read up to this point, then I thank you for using you precious time to enjoy my story and I wish you luck with residency and your future endeavours. And if you are a parent who is freaking out about the thought of your kid going to school in the Caribbean, then rest assured that I survived and everyone I know survived too. As parents, the best thing you can do for your child is be supportive, encouraging, understanding and of course send your child care packages! And for everyone else who read this – Thank you!

Dr. V

The amazing French tightrope walker Philip Petit once said, "you must first dream the dream and then build upon it". We all have dreams for ourselves and many of us set about making those dreams real. Others can't find the courage to make the leap into the unknown forced to remain lifelong spectators haunted by the "what ifs" of life. My strong message to anyone wanting to build their dream is jump and worry about the landing later. When you consider that RUSM now has well over 10,000 doctors practicing all over North America, you can see that if 10,000 people can jump and land safely, then you can too. You simply have to summon the courage and go!

Do I have regrets? Not really a regret, but rather a wish that I had done one thing differently. I wish in hindsight that I had had a mentor prior to applying to Canadian medical school. A mentor would have surely counselled me to apply to more than one medical school. I only applied to MUN, which was a big mistake as it limited my opportunities considerably. There are 17 medical schools across the country, and as a Canadian citizen, you can apply to all of them. Only applying to MUN was a big mistake in that regard. I don't dwell on that decision, but I share it so that others can learn from it.

Having said that, my journey through the jungle was a once in a lifetime, life-altering experience that I wouldn't trade for anything. It changed me forever. You learn to live independently away from home in a third-world country where every day can feel like a chore. You learn mostly about yourself and how much you can push the boundaries toward excellence. Most importantly, you learn to believe in you through isolation and self-reflection. You have the opportunity to meet people from all over the world and make life-long friends with people who share your common dream of being a Doctor.

You also gain a deeper appreciation for your family and in those many quiet moments, you come to realize how much you miss and love them every day. You also learn to rely on others both in the study groups and in your personal friendships. You learn to live a Spartan life, as the things we take for granted in North America are often scarce. You learn to help people who are less fortunate than you. I even met a family on the island who became my family; I stay in touch with them often and help when I can. It is a beautiful thing to be in the service of others; after all, isn't that what a Doctor is trained to do?

I am very grateful to have matched at the University of Ottawa in the Neurology program. I am surrounded by incredible teachers and colleagues in a very nurturing environment. I feel blessed and fortunate every single day. It was my top choice and I was theirs. Who could ask for more?

My take away message for the readers of this book who are considering medical school in the Caribbean is simple:

If you want it, go get it.
Only YOU know if you want it.

Is it hard?
Yes it is, but what in life is easy?

Can you do it?

Yes you can.

Will you be forever changed?
Yes you will.

Is the dream possible?
More than you know right now.

Go to the edge of the cliff.

Now jump...

And remember... You are not alone.

For those now going through the process: be strong, be patient and be kind. Those three things will never steer you wrong.

And always be focused and never get distracted by rabbit tracks when you are hunting elephants.

If you see a fellow student struggling offer a helping hand for as the old saying goes:

"The ones you meet going up the ladder are the same ones you meet on the way back down."

This is your time to shine and only you can rise to the occasion.

Dr. H

It's funny that when you finish the process, reach your goal and look back on the process, you forget the difficult times. I'm sure this would be different if I hadn't matched to Toronto. Don't get me wrong, I do remember the hardship I went through, but for some reason I don't have much to complain about. It was a choice that I had made and I was ready to deal with all the hardship that came with it.

Would I do it again? In a heartbeat if it meant that I would get to do what I do today, which is help and cure patients. Was it hard? I don't think anyone, but those who have gone through the process would understand what it was like. But in a way, I think the process made me a better person, a better physician. I know that I can deal with anything and everything and I will get through it. Going to school on an island with just the bare necessities, you realize that you can do without a lot of things. I have been exposed to different pathology, cases, health care systems, and living conditions from my travels during my four years of medical school. I have made wonderful lifelong friends through this journey.

Would I do anything differently? Yes, I would probably study harder during my undergraduate studies to make sure that my chances of getting in were higher. But, in a way, I don't regret the route that I took to get me to where I am today. In the process, I learned about myself, I was able to live alone and become independent. I met friends who are very dear to my heart and who are now my colleagues.

If you believe that medicine is for you and that it is your calling, then look at different options that will allow you to reach your goal. There isn't one route that fits everyone. Everyone that I have met reached his or her goals through different routes. The routes we take make us unique. Work hard during medical school. What you learn is the basis of your knowledge that you will come back to very often. When it comes to studying for exams, put everything you have forward to make sure you do really well. During rotations, don't be afraid to volunteer to do procedures, pick up more patients and do more work. Always ask for feedback and ways you can improve yourself. No one is perfect and there is always room for improvement in every one of us.

The most important thing of all is to pick your support group and your safety net because these will be the people that you will repeatedly come back to for support whether it is after encountering a difficult patient, a supervisor, or a hard exam. They will remind you that you are great at what you do and highlight what you have achieved; this will give you the strength to move forward. I don't think I could have done this process without my support group (my parents, siblings, my spouse, and my friends).

Lastly, try to enjoy life at each step in the process. To live a balanced life you need to have hobbies or sports that will allow you to relieve stress.

Overall this was the best decision I made for myself. I don't regret anything. The extra hours, the sleepless nights, the cries and frustrations with the process was all well worth it considering where I am today. I've finished my Family Medicine residency and currently enrolled in a Hospitalist Fellowship at University of Toronto.

Dr. R

Match day was rough. I didn't know what to do with myself. I was in Toronto and living back with my parents. I was a nervous wreck. I couldn't eat, couldn't sleep. At this point I felt desperate. All I wanted was to match; I didn't care if it was in California, Michigan or Zimbabwe (nom I didn't apply to programs in Africa). Big town or small – I was open to it all at this point.

I was overwhelmed and I am sure I drove all those around me crazy with hypothetical situations of me not matching and therefore having to move to Argentina to sell juice on the beach (in retrospect, my backup plan doesn't seem too bad). I felt insecure, alone and after I submitted my rank list, I was no longer in control; I felt helpless. So I escaped my parents' home, stayed at a friends place downtown, took a bunch of sleeping pills the night before (stop judging) and awoke the next day and kept refreshing and refreshing my Gmail screen. I was dizzy sitting on that leather couch with sunshine pouring into the 11th floor apartment near Bathurst and College. And finally, my fate arrived in black and white. Everything I had worked my entire life towards was now sitting in my Gmail inbox. Did I breathe before opening the email? Did I even have the capacity to think? I don't remember much. There it was right in front of my eyes as I sat alone in my friend's apartment "Congratulations, you have matched". Finally, all the pieces of my life started to fall into place.

I called my mom crying. Tears of joy and also feeling ashamed of the crazy anxiety I had put her through. She apparently had so much confidence in me she already knew I matched. What would I do without her?

Back in the day, the match was slightly more complicated than it is now. First, you match and two days later you get the program you matched to sent to you by email. At this point, I didn't care. I matched. That was that. I was going to be a doctor. Was I ready? To be honest I don't really think any of us are. We all have these preconceived judgments of what being a doctor is, what residency is like and where we are going. Residency was tough. Let's not pretend it wasn't. I worked in an 800-bed hospital in East LA. The patients were rough, the nurses were rough, the doctors were rough. I was consistently overwhelmed, but my skin is now thicker than ever. I met the good, the bad and the ugly (and I am not talking about my patients). Fierce competition for fellowship, strict rounding times, angry attendings (one attending even took the time to sit me down and tell me that as a female physician I have to be more assertive and learn to choose my words carefully; no more "likes" drizzled in my sentences - that definitely killed a part of my soul), bitchy nurses, long hours, high expectations, getting lost in a sea of residents with few people who know your name. It is a time in my life that taught me so much about human nature, dedication and trying you're hardest to live in the moment. Just when I thought medical school was the worst, I realized residency was harder. Just when you think things are hard, they get harder, and you push through.

But this path I am on is not done yet. The career is unique in that we are always forced to learn, grow, and interact with those during their lowest times. I learned about death, dying, disease, working with others in high-stress situations. There are not too many professions where this can be accomplished and there are not too many people who wish to deal with this.

Residency is like the sea: big, rough, full of up and downs, but ultimately beautiful.

"Reality is Wrong, Dream are for real" - Tupac Shakur

I am living my dream and I truly hope that you can live yours too. I must say the path was hard and there were many times (and late night phone calls to my mother) where I wanted to just give up and do nothing, but as I sit here after a 12-hour shift, I wouldn't go back and change it. Don't expect the road to be easy, don't except your friends and family to ever understand, and don't expect your patients to understand. I feel lucky to have been able to achieve my dream and will forever keep striving to be the best physician possible. Thank you for allowing me to share my journey with you.

APPENDIX I

DOMINICA

Short Name:Dominica
Capital City:Roseau
Languages:English, French Patois
Currency:Eastern Caribbean Dollar (XCD)
Exchange Rate:USD 1 : XCD 2.7169
Economy:Agriculture-based

Geography
Region:Eastern Caribbean
Location:Between Guadeloupe to the north and Martinique to the south
Latitude:15° 20' N
Longitude:61° 22' W
Surface Area:751 km2 (289.5 sq mi)
Highest Peak:Morne Diablotin - 1730 m (4,747 ft)
Climate:Humid tropical marine, little seasonal variation between the wet and dry season; high rainfall during the wet season.

Population
Population:69, 625 (2006 estimate)
Ethnic Groups:Black, Mixed, Amerindian (Caribs), White, Others
Religions:Roman Catholic, Seventh Day Adventist, Pentecostal, Methodist, Baptist, Anglican, Other

Government
Political Independence:November 3, 1978 (from United Kingdom)
Political System: Parliamentary Democracy
Head of State:President: His Excellency, Dr. Nicholas J. O. Liverpool, D.A.H. (October 2, 2003)
Head of Government:Prime Minister: Honorable Roosevelt Skerrit (January 8, 2004)
Elections:Last General Election - December 18, 2009
Next General Election - Constitutionally due by February 2015

MY NOTES

APPENDIX II
(from Carms website)
CaRMS

Returning to Canada
As a Canadian studying medicine outside of North America, you are not alone. The number of Canadians studying abroad (CSAs) has grown exponentially since 2000 and today approximately 130 schools in almost 30 countries have Canadian students enrolled in medicine. But while more than 90 per cent of CSAs want to return to Canada for postgraduate training, it can be a difficult journey.

When applying for residency training in Canada, CSAs are considered international medical graduates (IMGs) and enjoy no special privileges in a highly competitive Canadian matching process. In the past few years there has been a dramatic increase in the number of IMGs applying for residency positions in Canada and this increase is largely due to more Canadians studying medicine at international schools.

For a closer look at the numbers and success rates of Canadians returning to Canada after studying medicine abroad, you can check out the 2010 report on Canadian students studying medicine abroad.

The competition is stiff, but there are several ways you can prepare for entering a CaRMS residency match. First explore the more detailed content throughout CaRMS.ca.

CaRMS website: www.CaRMS.ca

MY NOTES

APPENDIX III
(from MCC website)

PHYSICIANS APPLY

All MCC-Online and PCRC-Online accounts and their contents have been moved to the new physiciansapply.ca system. MCC-Online and PCRC-Online have been deactivated. Instead of using two separate accounts, candidates can now log into their physiciansapply.ca account to:

- Submit requests for source verification of medical credentials issued outside of Canada
- Share medical credentials stored in the MCC Physician Credentials Repository
- Apply for MCC examinations
- View examination results and share them with registered medical organizations
- Apply for medical registration to an increasing number of medical regulatory authorities over the next 24 months (coming soon)
- To accompany the launch of the new system, the MCC has also launched a revamped version of its main website, mcc.ca.

Candidates can now activate their accounts by clicking “Login”.

physiciansapply.ca should be accessed using the following web browsers:

- Google Chrome
- Firefox
- Safari
- Internet Explorer 8 or 9
  If you have upgraded to the newer Internet Explorer (IE) 10, you may experience some difficulties. Activating “Compatibility view” under “Tools” in your IE10 browser might help.

Otherwise, it is recommended that you access physiciansapply.ca using another web browser.

The new system is not designed to be accessed through a mobile device at this time. A tablet-compatible version of the system will be available in the near future.

Accessing physiciansapply.ca for the first time:

Candidates should use their MCC-Online or PCRC-Online username and password to log into physiciansapply.ca for the first time. Candidates who have forgotten their MCC-Online and/or PCRC-Online user name and password should contact the Service Desk at 613-520-2240. Candidates who have taken MCC examinations in the past before online access was available and have never created a user account should also contact the MCC Service Desk at 613-520-2240.

New users (did not have an MCC-Online or PCRC-Online account, and have never taken an MCC examination) – can create a physiciansapply.ca account by clicking on Create an account on the physiciansapply.ca login page.

Once you log in, your account will need to be initialized. This process may take a bit of time to complete.

Formatting and usability at launch:

Candidates may experience some formatting and usability issues, including:

- The candidate's photo/signature will not be visible on his or her physiciansapply.ca account dashboard.
- The "Create a new message" link on the right-hand (third) panel of the dashboard is not functional; candidates must use the link in the middle (second) panel to send a new message to the MCC.

- Some document status icons may be incorrect. Please ignore the icons, such as a checkmark or an x. The written status, beside the icon, will be valid.
- For candidates logging into the system through inscriptionmed.ca (the French portal) – some labels, headings and help text incorrectly appear in English when they should be in French.
- The MCC will continue to work as quickly as possible to fix these issues.

For candidates from international medical schools who had documents verified and stored through MCC-Online:

Certain documents that were previously stored in candidates' MCC-Online account may not appear in their new account. These documents have been transferred to the candidate's new account, however an MCC staff person must review the data associated with the document before the candidate is able to view it.

Candidates applying for an MCC examination should first check their physiciansapply.ca account to see if they are able to view their medical degree/diploma in their list of documents. If they cannot see it, they should contact the MCC Service Desk and the MCC will make their document(s) visible in their account as soon as possible. Candidates should also contact the MCC if they need to share with another organization credential documents that were stored in MCC-Online and that they cannot see in physiciansapply.ca.

Contact information:

We thank you for your understanding during this period of transition. Should you have any questions or concerns, please contact the Service Desk:

mcc.ca/contact-us/
Telephone: 613-520-2240
Fax: 613-248-5234
Email: service@mcc.ca
MY NOTES

APPENDIX IV
(From govenrment of Canada website)

NEXUS PROGRAM

The NEXUS alternative inspection program has been completely harmonized and integrated into a single program. NEXUS members now have crossing privileges at air, land, and marine ports of entry. Under the Western Hemisphere Travel Initiative, the NEXUS card has been approved as an alternative to the passport for air, land, and sea travel into the United States for US and Canadian citizens.
The NEXUS program allows pre-screened travelers expedited processing by United States and Canadian officials at dedicated processing lanes at designated northern border ports of entry, at NEXUS kiosks at Canadian Preclearance airports, and at marine reporting locations. Approved applicants are issued a photo-identification, proximity Radio Frequency Identification (RFID) card. Participants use the three modes of passage where they will either present their NEXUS card or have their iris scanned and make a declaration.

U.S. Customs and Border Protection (CBP) and Canada Border Services Agency (CBSA) are cooperating in this venture to simplify passage for pre-approved travelers.

What Are The Benefits Of NEXUS?
Individuals approved to participate in NEXUS receive an identification card that allows them to:

- Receive expedited passage at NEXUS-dedicated lanes, airport kiosks, and by calling a marine telephone reporting center to report their arrival into the United States and Canada; and
- Cross the border with a minimum of customs and immigration questioning
- Use of Global Entry kiosks

NEXUS applicants only need to submit one application and one fee. Applicants may apply on-line via the CBP Global On-Line Enrollment

System (GOES) Web site. (GOES) Qualified applicants are required to travel to a NEXUS Enrollment Center for an interview. If they are approved for the program at that time, a photo identification card will be mailed to them in 7-10 business days. NEXUS allows United States and Canadian border agencies to concentrate their efforts on potentially higher-risk travelers and goods, which helps to ensure the security and integrity of our borders.

How Do I Apply?
Applications can be submitted using the CBP on-line application system, Global On-Line Enrollment System (GOES), or to one of the Canadian Processing Centers (CPC), along with photocopies of their supporting documentation and the US $50 or CN $50 application-processing fee. (GOES)

For NEXUS toll-free information (U.S. and Canada) call 1-866-NEXUS 26 (1-866-639-8726).

(06/05/2009)

MY NOTES

APPENDIX V

RUSM PROGRESS FLOW CHART FOR CANADIAN STUDENTS - SEMESTERS 1-10

Foundations of Medicine STEP 1
AICM Cores Physicians Apply Step 2 CS Step 2 CK MCCEE NAC Electives Statement of Need Health Canada

MY NOTES

APPENDIX VI
VISAS
(from the US government website)

Canadian medical students can be admitted to the U.S. for clinical clerkships or observer-ships on a B1 visa because they are not receiving any sort of salary related to these activities.

B1 visas are issued at the student's Canada/U.S. point of entry; however, be sure to get the paperwork needed from RUSM beforehand.

There are only two types of U.S. visas under which International Medical Graduates (IMGs) can be admitted into the U.S. for post-graduate medical training: J-1 Exchange Visitor and H1b Specialty Worker. Canadian citizens must apply for J1 or H1b visas in their home province or city of residence.

The J-1 Visa Waiver Program was put into effect in an effort to improve access to healthcare for residents of underserved areas in the U.S., and permits the Immigration and Naturalization Service (INS) to waive the foreign residency requirement in exchange for an agreement with an IMG who has completed medical training in the U.S. and who has agreed to practice primary care for at least three years in a federally designated health professional shortage or medically underserved area.

J-1 visas (which are good for the duration of training or up to seven years, whichever is more applicable) can only be sponsored by the ECFMG, which requires passage of USMLE Steps 1 and 2 (CK and CS), in addition to all other educational requirements as specified by the ECFMG. You are required to obtain a statement of need from Health Canada (www.hc-sc.gc.ca). In order to obtain the Statement of Need, you must take the MCCEE exam. While the requirements for being able remain in the U.S. after training with a J-1 visa are not as onerous as those associated with the H1b; the overall process may require the services of a lawyer, which can generate additional fees.

H1B visas are good for three years after issue and can be extended for an additional three years, after which an IMG needs to leave the U.S. for at least one year before being able to return and work on an H1b visa again. To obtain an H1b visa, U.S. government requirements must be fulfilled and the applicant must have taken and passed USMLE steps 1 through 3. The USMLE Step 3 cannot be taken until you have graduated from medical school. Keep in mind that most U.S. hospitals will not accept medical residents for training on H1b visas because of the extensive amount of paperwork involved.

MY NOTES

APPENDIX VII

CARMS APPLICATION SAMPLE TIMELINE (from the Carms website)

Applicant Timetable - First Iteration
Timetable for the first iteration of the 2012 R-1 match

NOTE: Milestones are CaRMS-recommended dates that you should follow to ensure you are using your time well and allotting enough time to complete the next phase thoroughly. These are not deadlines; they are merely guidelines that are proven to keep you on track throughout the match cycle. The five milestones in this timetable are: extra documents/transcripts expected at CaRMS milestone (October 28); submission of electronic application milestone (November 10); program selection milestone (November 16); letter of reference milestone (November 18); and document assignment milestone (November 23).

August 10, 2011 (12:00 ET) Online request for registration opens
September 2, 2011 Program descriptions updates complete
September 6 to 7, 2011 Applicant Webstation (AWS) access token distribution begins
September 7, 2011 (12:00 ET) Applicant Webstation (AWS) opens
October 12, 2011 (12:00 ET) Program selection opens
October 28, 2011 Extra documents/transcripts expected at CaRMS Milestone*
*This is the first milestone in the CaRMS first iteration timetable.
November 10, 2011 Application submission milestone
November 16, 2011 Program selection milestone
November 16, 2011 MSPR arrival - All Medical Student Performance Records (MSPRs) are due at the CaRMS office on this date.
November 18, 2011 Letter of reference milestone
November 23, 2011 Document assignment milestone
November 25, 2011 (17:00 ET) to December 1, 2011 (12:00 ET) AWS closed
December 1, 2011 (12:00 ET) File review begins

January 21 - February 12, 2012 National interview period
February 2, 2012 (12:00 ET) Rank order list (ROL) period begins
February 2, 2012 (12:00 ET) Request for registration closes
February 3, 2012 (12:00 ET) Late request for registration opens
February 15, 2012 (12:00 ET) Program ROL deadline
February 21, 2012 (16:00 ET) Applicant ROL Deadline

Note: Please check the CaRMS website for up-to-date info: www.carms.ca/eng/r1_1stIteration_e.shtml.

Tuesday, March 6, 2012 (12:00 ET) MATCH DAY

MY NOTES

APPENDIX VIII

HEALTH CANADA - STATEMENT OF NEED (from the Government of Canada website)

Statements of Need are issued by Health Canada, on behalf of provincial and territorial ministries of health, to medical graduates to assist them to obtain a J-1 Visa to enter the United States to pursue postgraduate medical training.

A Statement of Need is one of a number of requirements of the Exchange Visitor Sponsorship Program (EVSP), Educational Commission for Foreign Medical Graduates (ECFMG) that must be met before a J-1 Visa can be issued.

Below you will find a description of the program as well as instructions to apply for a Statement of Need.

Who issues Statements of Need in Canada?
What is a J-1 Visa?
How do I apply for a J-1 Visa?
What is a Statement of Need?
Who is eligible for a Statement of Need?
How do I apply for a Statement of Need?
What category should I use to apply for a Statement of Need?
Where do I submit my application?

Where do I submit my application?
Please submit all required documents to the Program Administrator, Health Canada. It is your responsibility to ensure all required documents are submitted. Complete packages are recommended and email is preferred. Certified and notarized documents cannot be submitted by facsimile.

Please submit your application by one of the following methods.

a. email (preferred)
b. courier
c. regular mail

d. facsimile (except notarized documents)

Email Address: j1visa@hc-sc.gc.ca
Subject: Application for Statement of Need, "Your Name"

Address for Mail and Courier:
Program Administrator
Statement of Need / J-1 Visa Program
Health Human Resources Policy Division
Strategic Policy Branch
Health Canada
Jeanne Mance Building, Address Locator 1918C
200 Eglantine Driveway
Tunney's Pasture, Ottawa Ontario, K1A 0K9

Telephone: 613 952 1912

Facsimile Address:
Program Administrator
Statement of Need / J-1 Visa Program
Health Human Resources Policy Division
Facsimile: 613 948 8081

When should I submit my application?

How long will it take to process my application?

Where does Health Canada send the Statement of Need?

I already have a Statement of Need - what do I do if I wish to change my specialty, change my location or undertake additional training?

Where can I get information on medical licensure in a province or territory in Canada?

How can I get help with finding employment in Canada?

What is the consent form for recruitment purposes?

What if I already have J-1 Visa sponsorship with another country?

Who do I contact for additional information?

MY NOTES

MY NOTES

APPENDIX IX

YEARS REQUIRED FOR CANADIAN SPECIALITIES

FAMILY MEDICINE	2 YEARS
INTERNAL	4 YEARS
GENERAL SURGERY	5 YEARS
EMERG5	5 YEARS
ANASTHESIOLOGY	5 YEARS
CARDIAC SURGERY	6 YERAS
THORASIC SURGERY	5 YEARS
DERMATOLOGY	5 YEARS
RADIOLOGY	5 YEARS
NEUROLOGY	5 YEARS
NEUROSURGERY	6 YEARS
OBGYN	5 YEARS
ORTHO	5 YEARS
PEDS	4 YEARS
MEDICINE REHAB	5 YEARS
UROLOGY	5 YEARS

MY NOTES

APPENDIX X
(from the NRMP website)

THE USA MATCH: NRMP

APPLICANTS

Registration for an ***NRMP*** Match requires logging in to the R3 system and completing the eleven-step registration process. The purpose of those steps briefly is described below:

- Select a Match: Identify in the ***R3*** system the Match for which you want to register.
- Participant Type: Indicate the type of medical school attended and citizenship status. Applicants in the Main Residency Match® also enter their expected date of graduation from medical school.
- Demographic Form: Provide basic profile information. Some applicants also are prompted to provide information such as USMLE® ID or NBOME® ID.
- Note. Profile information can be updated at any time during the Match process. Email addresses and phone numbers must remain current in the ***R3*** system to ensure receipt of important reminders, notices, and Match results from the NRMP.
- Login Credentials: Create a username and password to access the ***R3*** system.
- Match Participation Agreement: Read and electronically sign the legally binding agreement. The registration process is not complete until the Agreement has been signed.
- Payment: Pay the registration fee and the fee to participate as a couple, if appropriate, by credit card.

REGISTRATION INCLUDES THE FOLLOWING NRMP SERVICES:

- For the ***Main Residency Match***, processing of up to 20 different program ranks on the primary rank order list and up to 20 different program ranks on all supplemental rank order lists combined; each partner of a couple may process up to 30 unique programs on a primary rank order list and up to 30 unique programs on all supplemental lists combined.

- For the ***Specialties Matching Service***, processing of an unlimited number of ranks.
- Access to the List of Unfilled Programs (for qualifying applicants).
- Access to post-Match reports and data.

APPLICANT VERIFICATION

For the ***Main Residency Match***, the ***NRMP*** works with ***NRMP*** school officials to verify the credentials of students/graduates and Fifth Pathway enrolees/graduates of LCME-accredited medical schools, students/graduates of Canadian medical schools, and students/graduates of osteopathic medical schools.

Students/graduates of international medical schools (IMGs) must submit either:

- A notarized copy of a full and unrestricted license to practice medicine in a U.S. jurisdiction; or
- An Educational Commission for Foreign Medical Graduates (ECFMG®) candidate number. The ***NRMP***verifies with the ECFMG that applicants have completed the examination requirements for certification.
- For additional information on verification of credentials For Match eligibility, visit the ECFMG website.

All verifications must be completed by the Rank Order List Deadline in order to participate in the ***Main Residency Match***. An additional exchange between the ***NRMP*** and the medical schools and the ***NRMP*** and the ECFMG occurs after the Rank Order List Deadline to verify applicants' credentials for participation in the Match Week Supplemental Offer and Acceptance Program® (SOAP®).

MY NOTES

APPENDIX XI
(from the ERAS website)

ERAS

ERAS Support Services at ECFMG
The Association of American Medical Colleges (AAMC) developed the Electronic Residency Application Service (ERAS®) to allow medical school students and graduates to apply electronically for residency positions in accredited U.S. programs of graduate medical education.

Students and graduates of U.S. medical schools/programs are assisted in the ERAS process by the Dean's office at their medical schools. The Canadian Resident Matching Service (CaRMS) serves as the designated Dean's office for students and graduates of Canadian medical schools/programs who participate in ERAS. Since ERAS was established in 1996, ECFMG has served as the designated Dean's office for students and graduates of international medical schools, including Fifth Pathway participants, assisting these individuals with the ERAS application process for first- and second-year (PGY-1 and PGY-2) residency positions.

International medical students/graduates who apply to programs that participate in ERAS begin the application process by requesting an ERAS Token, a unique identification number, from ECFMG. The Token allows applicants to access AAMC's MyERAS website, where they can complete their residency applications, select the programs to which they will apply, and assign supporting documents to these programs.

As the designated Dean's office, ECFMG receives supporting documents for the ERAS application, such as Medical Student Performance Evaluations, medical school transcripts, letters of recommendation, and photographs from applicants, and their medical schools and letter writers. ECFMG then transmits these documents to the ERAS PostOffice. ECFMG also transmits to the ERAS PostOffice reports of an applicant's ECFMG certification status and, if requested by the applicant, USMLE transcripts. Once supporting documents have been received at the ERAS PostOffice, they can be downloaded by the programs to which the applicant has applied.

For more information on ERAS, visit the AAMC's ERAS website. For more information on ERAS Support Services at ECFMG, select the appropriate link below.

ERAS Support Services for Applicants
ERAS Support Services for International Medical Schools
ERAS Support Services for Letter Writers

MY NOTES

APPENDIX XII
(From Government of Ontario website)

RETURN OF SERVICE

What is ROS?
RETURN OF SERVICE AGREEMENT

The Ontario example:

International Medical Graduate Living in Ontario
As an international medical graduate (IMG) – someone who has completed his or her postgraduate residency training outside of Canada or the United States and whose medical degree is recognized by the World Health Organization (WHO) – navigating your way through licensing and certification in Ontario can be challenging, time-consuming and complicated.

Learn more about practice requirements, licensing and certification in Ontario and how HealthForceOntario Marketing and Recruitment Agency can help you achieve your goals.

Practice Requirements
The College of Physicians and Surgeons of Ontario (CPSO) regulates the practice of medicine in Ontario and issues certificates of registration to physicians to allow them to practice. An IMG who wishes to obtain an Ontario Certificate of Independent Practice through the CPSO must first meet the following registration requirements set out by the College:

Canadian citizenship, permanent resident status or authorization to work in Canada.
Passing results on the Medical Council of Canada (MCC) examinations.
Proof of language proficiency. This may involve taking the Test of English as a Foreign Language (TOEFL).

Completion of 1 year of postgraduate training or active medical practice in Canada, or completion of a full clinical clerkship at an accredited Canadian medical school.
Certification by either the Royal College of Physicians and Surgeons of Canada (RCPSC) or the College of Family Physicians of Canada (CFPC).

Licensing and Certification
This information is presented as a general guideline. Please visit the College of Physicians and Surgeons of Ontario (CPSO) website for the most up-to-date information regarding certification of registration. All information regarding licensure, examinations etc needs to be verified by contacting the appropriate regulatory and examining bodies.

An International Medical Graduate (IMG) can apply to Canadian Residency Matching Service (CaRMS) through the Postgraduate Year 1 (PGY1) pathway. CaRMS works in close cooperation with the medical education community, medical schools and students to provide an electronic application service and a computer match for entry into postgraduate medical training throughout Canada. Approximately 1,500 IMGs apply through CaRMS each year for approximately 200 residency positions in Ontario. Positions are granted to the most suitable candidates. Please visit the CaRMS website to view the full list of eligibility requirements. Because of the limited number of positions available each year, the process can be challenging and highly competitive. Only the most suitable candidates are selected based on the following:

Obtaining good scores on your Medical Council of Canada exams;
Professional practice experience;
Past performance in medical school;
Excellent communication (verbal and written) skills;
Reference letters;
Complete and professional CaRMS application; and
Your interview (if selected).
The above criteria does not guarantee a postgraduate medical training position (residency).

CFPC or RCPSC Certification

To obtain registration to practice in Ontario, physicians must have a specialty designation from either the College of Family Physicians of Canada (CFPC) or the Royal College of Physicians and Surgeons of Canada (RCPSC).

Find more information on receiving certification as a family medicine specialist from the CFPC.

Find more information on receiving certification as a specialist from the RCPSC.

Return-of-Service

An IMG who successfully completes a training position will be required to fulfill a 5-year Return of Service (ROS) contract in an underserviced community in Ontario. The ROS agreement is signed with the Ontario Ministry of Health and Long-Term Care.

MY NOTES

APPENDIX XIII
(From USMLE website)

PERSONAL STATEMENT

A part of every application process is the preparation of a personal statement. Generally speaking, residency programs will usually request a personal statement. A personal statement serves to complement and supplement your C.V. with a description of your qualifications and strengths in narrative form.

Sample from USMLE web:

Internal Medicine Personal Statement #1
Medicine encompasses numerous areas that I have always found intriguing. Becoming a physician is a lifelong dream that will fulfill both my personal and career goals. I feel privileged to have found a career that will allow me to accomplish all my aspirations; learning about the human body, helping people and educating them to take better care of their health.

Throughout my clinical rotations, I have found countless professors and physicians who were exceptionally willing to share their knowledge and experiences with me. I've also come to learn that being a teacher is a very critical part of being a physician. Education goes beyond attendings and their students/residents; it also carries over to patients. Explaining, communicating, and helping individuals understand and cope with their illness is an integral part of practicing medicine. One of my patients, whom we will call Mr. Smith, was diagnosed with a reentrant tachyarrhythmia. During my visit one morning, the cardiologist came to inform Mr. Smith of his findings. In addition, the doctor advised the patient to return so they can discuss the possibility of catheter ablation. I immediately sensed fear in Mr. Smith's eyes. After the cardiologist left the room, I asked him if he had any questions. He was silent for a while, and then asked, "So what is wrong with my heart?" I thoroughly and fundamentally explained what a PVC was and the procedures necessary to assist him. I answered all Mr. Smith's questions until he felt comfortable with the knowledge of his condition. I went back to see Mr. Smith on the day he was to be discharged and reiterated the importance of following up with the cardiologist. Prior to leaving, Mr. Smith looked at me with a smile on his face and said "Thank you for everything, you will make a great doctor". Mr. Smith's comment left me speechless and humbled. It was at that point I realized the importance of educating your patients.

Upon completion of my rotations, I felt most complete in Internal Medicine. I found Internal Medicine to be most rewarding at the end of the day. I found great enjoyment in the intellectual stimulation and working with adults. I have many attributes to contribute to internal medicine; I'm dedicated and loyal to my cause, I have great listening skills as well as interpersonal skills, I'm a critical thinker and problem solver. As a decisive thinker, I plan to use deductive reasoning to reach a diagnosis from the data obtained about a patient. Moreover, Internal medicine has much to offer in return such as the diversity of medical conditions and the comprehensive medical care over long periods of time. Furthermore, I find the challenges of treating a broad range of illness enjoyable and rewarding.

On a personal note, I feel that being a physician is a privilege and an honor that should not be taken lightly. The responsibility of caring for one's health is both significant and fulfilling. To treat an ill individual and nurse them back to health is awe-inspiring. I'm reminded of a quote that I once read which states that "medical education is not completed in medical school: it is only begun". Thus far, my journey has been most gratifying and has reached beyond all my expectations. I look forward to the challenges and endeavors to come. The road to medicine is not about the destiny but the journey itself and I look forward to that journey.

MY NOTES

APPENDIX XIV

INTERNATIONAL MEDICAL GRADUATE

Definition of an IMG
ECFMG and its organizational members define an international medical graduate (IMG) as a physician who received his/her basic medical degree or qualification from a medical school located outside the United States and Canada. The location of the medical school, not the citizenship of the physician, determines whether the graduate is an IMG. This means that U.S. citizens who graduated from medical schools outside the United States and Canada are considered IMGs. Non-U.S. citizens who graduated from medical schools in the United States and Canada are not considered IMGs.

MY NOTES

APPENDIX XV

BANKS THAT PROVIDE LINES OF CREDIT (LOCs) TO STUDENTS

(ALL INORMATION GATHERED BELOW IS AVAILABLE ON EACH BANK"s WEBSITE)

BMO – BANK OF MONTREAL

With competitive rates, Bank of Montreal offers a Professional or Medical Student Line of Credit which can be used for tuition, living and travel expenses while attending school. Students are encouraged to contact their local BMO branch directly to discuss the advantages of a banking relationship with BMO.

Professional or Medical Student Lines of Credit
Pursuing a professional designation demands focus. BMO Professional or Medical Student Lines of Credit let you stay focused on what's important—your studies.

- Borrowing designed for your specific program
- Easy access to funds – BMO debit card, Student Line of Credit MasterCard®*, write a cheque or visit any branch.
- No annual, monthly or ABM fees
- Free Student Line of Credit MasterCard access card let's you access your Line of Credit anywhere MasterCard is accepted
- Pay interest only on what you borrow while you're in school1 and for up to one year after graduation, followed by a gradually escalating repayment schedule
- Ask us about repayment plans for your program2
- As you pay down your balance (and monthly interest payments) you can keep borrowing up to your credit limit
- Optional Creditor Life and Disability/Disability Plus Job Loss Insurance

Available Credit Limit

Credit Limit Per Year	Total Maximum Credit Limit
$50,000	$200,000

1. Includes up to 2 years of specialty studies for Dentistry Professional Student Line of Credit and for Medical Student Line of Credit monthly interest payments applies to a maximum of 7 years of residency.
2. Applies only to Dentistry Professional Student Line of Credit and for Medical Student Line of Credit only. Certain conditions apply. Visit your local branch or call 1-877-CALL-BMO for complete details.
   * A co-signer may be required. Subject to credit availability and verification of identity.

Are You Eligible?

You must:

- Be a Canadian citizen or landed immigrant
- Be enrolled in a Canadian or non-Canadian post-secondary school or university
- Meet BMO's usual credit criteria

For More Information

Visit: Bank of Montreal website

Call: (780) 408-0123 and speak with Kim Wolf

Email: Kim Wolf

NATIONAL BANK OF CANADA

National Bank of Canada feels that, as a full-time student and future health sciences specialist, you are entitled to a financial package that includes privileges on a range of products and services.

The Student Line of Credit is a convenient and flexible solution for:

- Financing all your annual tuition and education-related expenses.
- Designed as a regular Chequing account: you can access your funds at any time via Client-Card purchases, Electronic Banking Solutions or cheques.

Main advantages:

- Credit limit established according to your needs
- Prime rate + 0.75%
- No monthly administrative fees
- Funds instantly accessible at all times
- Interest calculated only on principal used
- Option of deferring principal payments for up to 12 months after completed studies, within credit limit. However, interest accrues during that period. Only interest and insurance premium payments (if applicable) must be made monthly.
- Subject to credit approval from National Bank of Canada.
- The prime rate means the annual variable interest rate published by National Bank of Canada from time to time and used by the Bank to determine the interest rates on demand loans granted by it in Canadian dollars in Canada.
- Subject to credit approval by National Bank of Canada. A guarantor who satisfies the Bank's criteria may be required. The annual amount is base on your personal budgetary requirements. Gradual limit increases are possible. Certain specific conditions may apply. The minimum monthly payment is limited to monthly interest charges.
- Examples of interest charges for a 30-day period at the rate applicable on March 11th 2009:

	Average Balance	Average Balance
Annual Interest Rate	$500.00	$3,000.00
Prime Rate = 2.50%	$1.03	$6.16

For more information regarding the advantages and conditions of the National Bank's Student Line of Credit, please visit advisors at the National Bank branch nearest you.
Call: 1-866-987-1031
Visit: National Bank's website
Email: National Bank of Canada Wealth Management

RBC – ROYAL BANK OF CANADA

RBC Plan for Medical & Dental Students provides flexible financing options, convenient banking services and the one to one attention you deserve.

RBC Medical & Dental Student Specialists will be your point of contact, bringing you banking, credit and investment advice, all in one place. They will be there when you need them, for advice, support and access to financial solutions created, just for you, through the ease and convenience of a single relationship.

Student Line of Credit
RBC offers you the freedom to borrow what you need, when you need it:

- A $200,000 Student Line of Credit1 at prime, with no restrictions on how much you can borrow annually.
- Option to defer principal payments until 12 months after completion of residency. Students who are not required to complete residency have the option to defer principal payments until 12 months after graduation.

Student Banking
Student Banking is free while you are in medical or dental school. Convenient student banking is designed to save you money and make it easier to fit your banking needs into your schedule. The following free services are included:

- Deposits, withdrawals and transfers2
- 12 drafts and money orders per year
- Automated transfers between RBC Royal Bank accounts

- Access to your account 24/7 via Online, Telephone, Interact† direct payment and ATM banking
- Commission fee on Amex traveller cheques3
- An RBC Rewards VISA* Gold card with no annual fee1** - Earn one RBC Rewards point for every $2 spent on the card - Minimum credit limit of $5,000
- Discount on Royal Bank of Canada car loan interest rates A discount of 1% off the standard car loan rate1

1. Subject to credit approval
2. Excludes Interac, PLUS and/or convenience fees from other Financial Institutions' ATMs.
3. Applies to single signature only † Trademark of Interac Inc. Used under license. * Registered trademark of VISA International Service Association. Used under license. ** I understand if I do not qualify for an RBC Rewards Visa Gold card you may consider my application for an RBC Rewards Visa Classic card with no annual fee. ® Registered trademark of Royal Bank of Canada. TM Trademark of Royal Bank of Canada. ® RBC and Royal Bank are registered trademarks of Royal Bank of Canada.

Application Process

Students must provide:

1. Confirmation that you are enrolled at a post-secondary international educational institution and pursuing a medical degree.
2. An estimate of your education costs (including tuition, supplies, fees, accommodations, food, travel and other qualified expenses.)
3. A list of your financial resources (including savings, bursaries, summer employment, etc.)

Allow 5 business days from time of application for review, approval and funding of line.

For More Information

Call: 1-800-769-2511 to talk to a Credit Specialist and apply by phone.

Visit: Royal Bank of Canada Website
Branch Locator: Royal Bank of Canada Branch Locator

TD CANADA TRUST

TD Canada Trust understands that higher education doesn't come cheap. Being a student, you already know that. To give you a hand with your expenses, TD Canada Trust customized their Student Lines of Credit so that you can get the help you need to cover the cost of such things as tuition, books and living expenses.
With a TD Canada Trust Student Line of Credit, you can have access to the money you need, when you need it and use it for whatever you want. But you'll also get much more:

- Pay no monthly or annual fees.
- Get a competitive interest rate, equal to TD Prime plus a variance rate. Good news: the variance rate doesn't increase after you graduate!
- Withdraw any amount (up to your approved credit limit).
- Pay interest-only monthly payments for up to 12 months after your finish school.
- Enjoy low monthly payments after the interest-only grace period, with up to 20 years to repay.
- Access your money through Green Machine ABMs, Interac Direct Payment, EasyWeb Internet banking, EasyLine telephone banking, cheques and at any TD Canada Trust branch.

Lines of Credit
Professional students enjoy all the benefits of a standard Student Line of Credit with higher credit limits that are tailored to the unique needs of tomorrow's professionals.

TD Canada Trust Line of Credit Life Insurance
Should something happen to you, TD Canada Trust Line of Credit Life Insurance can help protect your family from outstanding debt. Since your premiums are calculated automatically based on your revolving credit balance, you pay for this valuable coverage only when you need it. And applying is easy.

Available when TD Canada Trust Student Line of Credit is programmed on your Access Card. Fees may apply.

For More Information
Call: 1-866-222-3456 for more information or application on our Student Lines of Credit
Visit: TD Canada Trust's website
Read: Student Line of Credit FAQs

SCOTIA BANK

Scotia Professional® Student Plan (SPSP) is a customized professional banking program that provides solutions and and strategies to help you achieve your financial goals, now and in the future. Features include:

- A <u>Scotia Powerchequing® Account</u> with all monthly service charges waived as long as you're in school and up to twelve months after graduation or completion of residency/articling. Included is an Overdraft Protection limit.
- A Scotia Professional Student Plan Line of Credit with the flexibility of no monthly payments - interest is simply added to your principal balance, while you're within your credit limit, for as long as you remain in school and up to twelve months after graduation or completion of residency/articling.
    - Included are free line of credit cheques, optional ScotiaLine® Protection insurance coverage, and convenient itemized statements.
- Access to your funds by cheque, in person or by phone, Internet, direct payment or Scotiabank automated banking machines.
- Your choice of:
    - No-Fee Scotia Moneyback® VISA* card with a $5,000 pre-approved limit; Disclosure statement - Read before you apply (40 kb) OR
    - No-Fee ScotiaGold® VISA* card with a $5,000 pre-approved limit. Disclosure statement - Read before you apply (40 kb)

- RSP Account RSP and self-directed RSP plan administration fees waived.

The Scotia Professional Student Plan has been designed for students, who are Canadian citizens or landed immigrants, enrolled in an academic program at a Canadian university leading to a professional degree in medicine, dentistry, veterinary medicine, chiropractic, optometry, pharmacy, law or joint law and MBA programs.

Apply Online
Apply now using our online application. If your academic program is not eligible for Scotia Professional Student Plan, you may wish to consider applying for a ScotiaLine® personal line of credit for students.

DISCLAIMER
All student loan information contained herein has been gathered from each lenders' website as of February 14 and is subject to confirmation by the lender directly.

- All loan programs listed are subject to revision as per applicable lender.
- All programs listed are subject the given lender's credit criteria.
- All lenders make final loan decisions

MY NOTES

CPSIA information can be obtained at www.ICGtesting.com
Printed in the USA
LVOW08s1616230414

382933LV00003B/677/P

9 781632 631213